*A nutrition expert e.
how this half-century old
science helped him to lose
over 100 lbs., and keep it off
for over a decade.*

zero resistance weight loss

how to lose weight naturally and fast

Matthew Good, MS, RD, LD

Good Health Industries
PO Box 4807
Austintown, Ohio 44515
www.elementsofgoodhealth.com

Ordering Information:

Regarding quantity sales, special discounts are available on bulk purchases by corporations, associations, and others. For details, contact the publisher at the address above.

ISBN: 978-1483970141

First Edition

Dedication

For my family. Without your support, nothing I have accomplished or ever will, the least of which being this book, would be possible.

Foreword

By Cindy Miketa

"Your enthusiasm excites me! And as for me "having my hands full" with you, let's face it; I went into a business of helping people lose weight. And on top of that, I am almost always their "last chance". My business is accepting challenges, but my reward, seeing someone accomplish their goals and being comfortable in their own skin, is an amazing feeling."

This was the response I received from Matt the very first day I emailed him about his services. His response made me feel like he was really interested in working with me and he was willing to see this through with me no matter what. Little did I know how right I actually was. This was the beginning of the end of my life in the world of dieting as I knew it.

I, like so many others, have tried every diet out there; losing and gaining, losing and gaining, as if all my efforts were destined to be in vain. I then received a postcard in the mail from Good Health Industries proclaiming to have a new take on weight loss, an advertisement touting "unparalleled support mechanisms to guarantee your weight loss goal." It was very intriguing, I must say; so intriguing that I held on to that postcard for almost a year before I decided to do something with it.

There I sat at my computer; an email that I wrote, addressed to info@elementsofgoodhealth.com, staring at my computer screen. It was a simple email, simply asking for more information on the services offered; nothing to take note of. I just couldn't decide whether to hit the "Send Message" or the "Delete Message" button and just forget about it. Thinking back to that day, maybe one of the reasons was because I wasn't sure if I was ready to make another commitment to a weight loss program. I had received plenty of eye-appealing advertisements throughout the years offering the "newest" and most "improved" methods of weight loss. But, I just kept getting drawn back to that postcard I received. With all this in mind, I guess it's not hard to defend why it took me so long to decide if this latest offer was worth my time and another commitment. Spoiler Alert! I hit the "Send Message" button. It was one decision I will never regret.

From the first moment that he personally answered my email, I knew there was something different about Matt and his services. In regards to my opening paragraph, I honestly did believe I was going to be a "challenge", because I did not think I could lose weight again. At 57 years old I had just about given up hope, surrendered to the thought that weight loss simply might be an impossibility for me. If you are reading this, I am sure that you have had a similar feeling of helplessness before. Yet, through the development of some personal health issues, I had a new reason to want to lose weight. The reality that if I did not do something now, make permanent lifestyle changes, I would be living the rest of my life in a lot of pain, and taking medication I wanted nothing to do with, must have been the push that I needed to get started and make that commitment. I found the strength to give it one last shot, and I honestly believe that this was my "last shot". Funny thing about that; Matt must have sensed it was my last shot as well. One of the first quirky sayings that Matt tends to spout off from time to time was "Welcome to the beginning of the last time you'll ever try to lose weight." It wasn't long before I was on my way to a new life. I always knew there was something more to losing weight other than "eat less, exercise more." Don't get me wrong, both of these things have their place, but that's just half the story. Think you're ready to hear the other half?

Through my first few months of working with him, Matt often asked me, "What is different this time than any other time you have tried to lose weight?" At first I didn't know what to say. I knew his method was working; after all, the weight was coming off at a faster pace than what I had been used to. My "dieter" mentality told me it was because I was eating right again and getting on my treadmill (which did have a lot to do with it). But something else was changing that took me a little longer to figure out; something that Matt was trying to get me to recognize the entire time. Something that I know now that each of his clients finds within themselves, that changes us from the inside out. I started realizing my whole attitude toward the "dieting life" was evolving. I was handling life's problems, both little and big, differently than I did before. For the first time in my life, I learned how to handle these issues without using food to solve my problems.

Remember when I said that eating right and exercise was only half of the story? Well, that other half is what makes Matt so special to those that know him and have had the pleasure of working with him. He's been in my shoes. He's been in your shoes. He knows the feeling of helplessness with food. Just look at the cover of this book; his "before and after" pictures prove that. I think of all those times that people would just pound it into my head that this whole dieting thing is mind over matter. "Just don't eat this or that. All that you need is willpower." But Matt validated what I had subconsciously wanted to believe all long. There had to be something more than willpower and just because I am on a diet does not mean that life will stop attempting to screw that up, and that's what Matt helped me to fix.

My epiphany came when that feared moment found its way into my life, when the weight loss began slowing down. The dreaded "plateau". However, for the first time in my life, I did not want to quit. I found myself even more motivated to do this or that to get the weight off; I wanted to work harder. Believe it or not, my treadmill became my new best friend; and did I ever hate that treadmill. I found myself messaging Matt, looking to him to verify what I thought I needed to do. Again he asked me, "What is different this time than any other time you have tried to lose weight?" I still had no response.

Matt is very good at asking his clients questions, already knowing the answer, and leading them to figure it out for themselves. Maybe that's a carryover from teaching aspiring Dietitians, as well. Having a hard time answering this one question, he gave me a book to read; this book.

That's when I knew the answer to Matt's' question. What was changing was not about how much weight I lost, but what I was gaining by losing the weight. I had always focused on the numbers, and when the numbers didn't reflect my efforts, I would throw in the towel and give up.

I was also a "weigh-a-holic", stepping on the scale every day. This caused a lot of stress and anxiety with me during my weight loss journey. So much so that I literally had to give up my scale and only weigh in once a month, which would be during my session with Matt. I had to realize it was not about numbers, even though that's what everyone, including myself, wants to believe; it is more about your personal goals, your accomplishments and how you feel about yourself. Think about the last time you lost weight. What is the first thing people say to you when it begins to show? "How much weight have you lost?" Sure it's a little rewarding. But just think how much better you would feel telling someone what you have gained by losing weight, not what you lost. I believe in myself so much more now than I have ever believed before.

So here I am, about a year and a half after receiving that postcard in the mail, and about nine months since I actually met Matt face to face. I have lost a great deal of weight. My "tight" clothes are loose. I have been able to reduce some of my medications. Don't get me wrong, all of these things are great. But let me tell you my answer to Matt's question, "What is different this time than any other time you have tried to lose weight?" I no longer live my life waiting for my weight loss attempt to fail; I live my life knowing that I will succeed.

My self-confidence is through the roof, because Matt's confidence in me put it there. There is an end to my journey this time. The weight will come off; and at that point, I will begin my new journey of keeping it off, and living a life doing things that I never thought would be possible again.

I am still a work in process; but the one thing I am not any more is a "challenge". I continue to work with Matt, and continue to learn more about myself every day. Most importantly, I continue to experience my "Zero Resistance Weight Loss".

If in the future you were to have the pleasure of seeing Matt speak or better yet, working with Matt personally, make no mistake. He will ask you "What is different this time than any other time you have tried to lose weight?" Your answer may very well be different from mine, and you may not have that answer right at your fingertips, but you can find that answer in the pages of this book.

Wishing all of you the very best of luck on your weight loss journey,

Cindy

Table of Contents

Introduction

If you have flipped to this Introduction, chances are that you are (1) standing in a book store, or have downloaded a "teaser" to the full-length eBook, trying to figure out if this book is something you are interested in, or, (2) have already purchased this book on a whim, or as a result of a suggestion from a friend or someone else of influence in your life, trying to find the motivation to engage in its content. I truly hope that it seems like I am reading your thoughts. I intend for the content of this book to operate as a precursor, or at least simultaneously to your thoughts as the book progresses. I want you to be thinking "This book must have been written just for me." Why on Earth would I attempt to take on such a challenge as an author? Well, I do not view it as a challenge. Through my years of teaching at the collegiate level, I have found it to be of exponential benefit to my students if I am able to lead them to deduce the correct answer, as opposed to simply handing it to them. I have since applied that method in my weight management practice with my clients. In full disclosure, I do not find this to be very difficult because you, my clients, and I are not that different; just as we are not that different from the millions of others who have struggled to lose weight at some time in their life. Bear with me while I briefly explain a little about myself.

I am a Registered Dietitian, with more than adequate formal education and training to be considered an expert and authority in the field of nutrition, especially in regards to weight loss. Now let's put that idea on the back burner for a moment. I do not wish to minimize the importance of formal education and experience, however I feel as if I can be of a greater service to you by sharing my personal experience, as well as professional, with a great deal of emphasis being placed on the former. In chronological order, I have eighteen years' experience living a life at what my mother would have so kindly referred to as being "big boned", being born into this world near ten pounds, and always staying true to that "high percentile" trend. Then came two years' experience when I perfected the art of unadulterated weight gain, blindly walking a path that led to me gaining well over one hundred pounds.

This was followed by a handful more years' experience suffering terrible failures at being the governance of my own health, accepting my fate of obesity. I then experienced spiteful success in reigning in my habits in regards to my body's weight. I continue to experience, and take note of the priceless events in my life, as well as such events of my client's lives. Throughout my extensive training, pricelessly coupled with personal experience, I have acquired one key attribute that I believe has allowed me the good fortune to comprehend the unrestricted veracity of obtaining a healthy weight; compassion. I have empathy for the overweight and obese; and please not mistake my use of the word empathy with sympathy. This is not to say that I "feel sorry" for what you or I have gone through. Rather, it is my empathy regarding that seemingly insurmountable process of weight loss that has assigned me the mission to spread the word of just how manageable losing weight can be. This empathy has allowed me to analyze the data of my years of professional and personal experiences, coming to formidable theory as to why I have been able to do what so many others find so difficult. It is this empathy that has driven me to dissect this theory into practical applications that each and every one of us can put into practice every moment of our lives. To be concise, the contents of this book will teach you how to lose weight using the exact methods that have helped me personally, as well as a collective of my personal clients, lose countless thousands of pounds, changing my life and theirs, moment by moment, ounce by ounce.

So, what can you expect from the pages in this book? Let me start by telling you what you should not expect. This book does not contain a specific diet to follow, nor does it contain medical advice pertaining to nutrition and diet. That type of information is widely available through an appointment with a Registered Dietitian, searches of credible websites offering information on well-balanced, calorically-restricted meal plans, or by simply turning on your favorite daytime television show that features medical advice. To be honest, the idea of another recount of well-balanced, calorically restricted diets to lose weight taking up the valuable real estate in this book irks me beyond belief. Our world contains such a wealth of information regarding weight loss, to reiterate it here would be a waste of your time and mine. What is truly troubling, with all of this information, and with widespread acknowledgement being paid to what is *not* working, as evidenced by the ever-rising obesity trend, there is very little attention being paid to changing the paradigm as to how we approach reigning in our waistlines. That is exactly what the content of this book offers; a new paradigm of weight management, starting with your mind.

I hope those last four words in the previous paragraph have not discouraged you from continuing with this book. It has been my experience that as soon as the idea of "self-improvement" or "self-help" comes into play, we immediately begin to associate the idea with hocus pocus, head-shrinking, or even witch craft. But rest assured, the theory behind this book, as well as the practical applications that are filling its pages, have been deciphered from classic self-improvement principles established by the pioneers, and world-renowned experts in the field, such as Maxwell Maltz, and Napolean Hill. .

At this point, I will close this introduction by issuing you a challenge. Should you have already decided that this book might be just what you are looking for, by all means, continue to read the text chapter by chapter, and implement its lessons that have worked for millions of people before you. Should you be finding yourself more apprehensive about continuing with this book, I ask you to honestly answer these simple questions.

Has your mental attitude or even a fleeting negative thought ever thwarted your weight loss attempt?

Have you ever made a single mistake on your diet plan, just to convince yourself that you are a failure?

Have you ever skipped a workout, either willingly, or a consequence of schedule conflict, and told yourself you are just too busy and you can start again on Monday?

Have you ever hit a weight loss plateau, becoming convinced that that is the weight you are intended to be stuck at?

Are you looking for someone who has experienced everything that you have, if not more, who is willing to share how to overcome these obstacles?

Do you feel as if you spend every minute of every day worried about losing weight?

If you answered yes to any of these question (and I know that you did), don't fret. But a particularly bothersome question is that last one; *"Do you feel as if you spend every minute of every day worried about losing weight?"* From a mathematical standpoint, we spend about two hours a day eating, and hopefully a half hour to an hour a day exercising, along with eight hours a day sleeping. That leaves us with roughly thirteen hours every day that we are *thinking* about losing weight. Thirteen hours every day that we are convincing ourselves to eat or not to eat, to exercise, or not to exercise, what to eat and how much of it to eat, how to exercise and how long to do it. That's over three-quarters of your day dedicated to your weight loss goals that exist only in your mind. So doesn't it make sense that by training your brain to easily handle these situations, your weight loss goals will become effortless, obtainable with Zero Resistance? Welcome to your Zero Resistance Weight Loss life.

How to Use this Book

I would love to tell you that simply by passively reading the following pages that you will be rewarded with some secret knowledge or super power that will make the act of losing weight completely effortless. Unfortunately, that is not the case. What this book does provide you with is invaluable information and practical applications to essentially "get out of your own way on the road to weight loss success."

Therefore, this book must be read in an active fashion. From chapter to chapter, section to section, page to page, concentrate on the message of the lesson you are learning. Reflect on whether the personal attributes being described are something that resembles personality characteristics that you embody. If so, practice with the tools provided to identify, eliminate, and replace these negative habits or characteristics with new, healthier ones.

Some of the concepts in this book are simple, while others being far more abstract; and abstract thoughts may not be absorbed at first glance. You may need to reread pages, or chapters, or the entire book before your light bulb turns on, and your "Aha" moment happens.

I am very happy to tell you that you do not have to walk this journey alone. While I would like to teach you everything that I know about losing weight, I would also like to learn everything that you know. Let's make this an active learning experience. By purchasing a copy of this book, you are now entitled to a wealth of tools far more powerful than any printed words. I have created a special *Member's Only* website, reserved for my private clients and now open to the readers of this book. Inside this membership site, you will find:

> ➤ A powerful social networking component designed specifically for one goal; losing weight. Our social network allows you to communicate with people who are trying to lose, or who have lost weight. With all the powerful functionality of popular social networking sites, you'll be "posting", "liking", "sharing", "following", and interacting your way to a smaller waistline!

> ➤ *Fitness University*; an ever-expanding library of credible information and useful videos that will put you on the fast track to your weight loss goal. This isn't about boring lectures, but practical and easily implemented strategies to make sure you are moving

towards your goal every minute of every day. For starters, you can begin by watching the eight-part video series that accompanies this book.

➢ A direct line of access to me, ready to answer your questions and provide you with guidance using the same techniques that afforded me the ability to lose over 100 lbs.

Unlocking this free, yet immensely powerful membership is easy. Just visit members.ElementsOfGoodHealth.com to sign up. My personal goal for developing this site is simple; I wanted to create a community of people all striving for the same thing, while sharing everything that I have learned in my personal journey to success. Imagine the powers that may be harnessed when people gather, all having that burning desire to achieve a healthy body that they are comfortable living their life in. Please, become a part of it.

I cannot think of any other ways to effectively communicate with you the priceless information that you hold in your hands. If you have other ideas, please let me know. Until then...

...Learn actively, implement quickly, and be on your path to Zero Resistance Weight Loss.

Chapter One

You, in a Nutshell

Throughout my years of experience, both professionally and personally, I have developed an ever-expanding comprehension of the importance of the mind concerning weight loss. Over time, I have realized that a well-balanced diet and well-designed exercise program are relatively useless; that is, if the mind isn't on board. After coming to this realization some time ago, I have professed this notion to my clients to be of the utmost importance. However, I now realize the injustice that I was a part of. Not because of the message itself, but because of the disorganization of my delivery of the information.

As mentioned in the Introduction, I am a student of the late Dr. Maxwell Maltz, the originator of the science of self-improvement, which he baptized as Psycho-Cybernetics. I owe a great deal of gratitude to a dear friend of mine, John Delserone, who suggested that I read Dr. Maltz's book, as he believed the message that I was attempting to spread paralleled much of what Psycho-Cybernetics encompasses. Yet, there were two key differences. One, while Dr. Maltz has provided millions of people a practical method of realizing their potential of becoming a superior version of themselves in a very broad sense, I was streamlining a similar theory into how these people could live a healthy life, in a body they were comfortable living it in. Two, my cognitive weight loss theories and applications resembled more of a muddled mess compared to the message Dr. Maltz ever-so eloquently delivered.

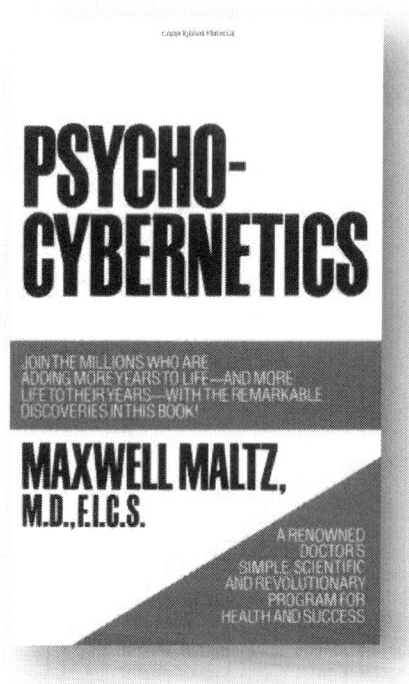

Figure 1. Psycho-Cybernetics, Dr. Maxwell Maltz

It is for these two reasons that I chose to write this book. I do not intend to reinvent the wheel, nor do intend to improve on it. What I do intend is to take that wheel, and put a new tire on it. The vehicle remains the same. The wheel remains the same. I would just like to make it more suitable for the conditions of your journey towards a specific goal; weight loss. I simply cannot improve on the science that Dr. Maltz has left us with; but what I can do, and view it is my duty to do, is to make his science fit into the weight loss equation. If you have ever read Dr. Maltz's Psycho-Cybernetics (and if you haven't, I highly recommend that you do), you will notice parallel's in his teaching, and that of my own. I have even gone to the extent of using the same terminology that he fashioned. I do this, not because of its simplicity and effortlessness, but because what he had developed over a half of a century ago is a science in and of itself, and deserves to be treated that way, terminology and all.

The Self-Image

Let us first lay the groundwork for how to accomplish weight loss with zero resistance. It all begins with the self-image. In essence, the self-image is life's paradigm. That is, it does not necessarily tell us where we go in life, but it does help to shape how we experience life's events. Each and every one of us has limitless potential. Since the idea of "limitless" or "infinite" is difficult for the human mind to comprehend, we impose on ourselves temporary limitations. I will refer to these as goals; as a goal, by definition, is something to be accomplished, an ending. This is the very meaning of the word is finite. Such as, if we complete X, Y, and Z, then we will reach our goal. However, that does not mean that life ends after reaching a goal. It simply means that a new goal must be set. This goal setting and accomplishment cycle is repeated over and over again throughout life, making our potential limitless and infinite. Goals, simply put, are our way of making infinite more understandable.

The Sort of Person I Am

No negative consequence should arise from setting temporary limitations on ourselves, such as goals, because the essence of a goal is something to be accomplished. The problem lies when (1) no goal is set, which we will discuss in later chapters, and (2), when we place false limitations on our potential through that of an ill-conceived self-image.

As you can see in Figure 2. The Self and the Self-Image, the self lies at the center, and is everything that you currently are; your conscious mind. Again, this self has unlimited, or infinite growth potential, afforded to us through such behaviors as goal setting. When you set a goal, there is no doubt it is born from a desire to better yourself in some way. The self-image acts like something of an invisible force field, temporarily dictating just how much potential the self has to grow, or just how likely you are to accomplish a goal. Many, many of us tend to let this invisible force, the self-image, close in on us, forcing us to believe in the false small area of growth that is able to be achieved, or our limited abilities to accomplish our goals. As Dr. Maltz would put it, the self-image mirrors "the sort of person I am." Ponder these general questions for a moment:

> *Can I wake up 30 minutes early for work as take a brisk walk?* If you answered "No", you might interpret LAZY as the sort of person you are.

> *Can I focus on eating smaller portions?* If you answered "No", you might interpret WEAK-WILLED as the sort of person you are.

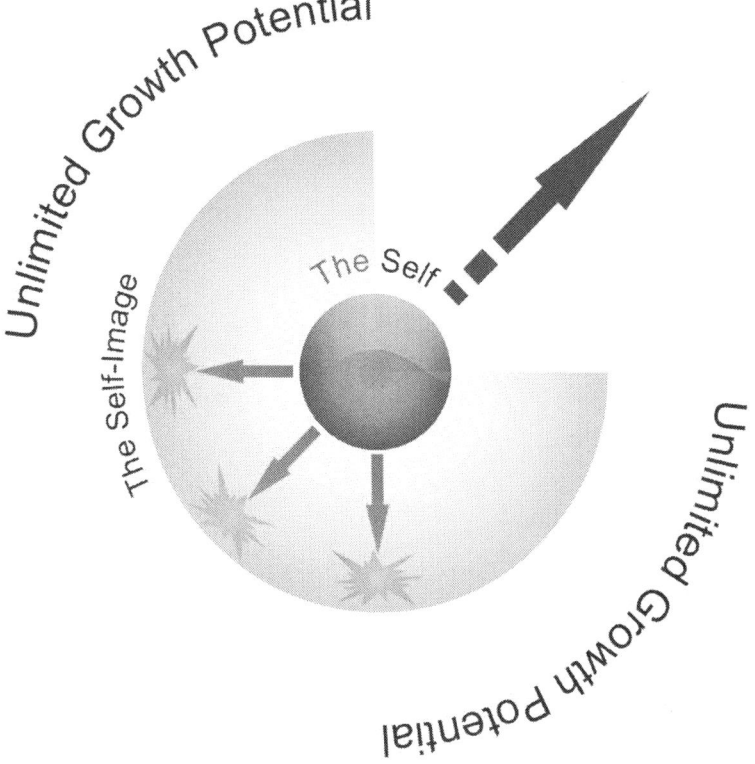

Figure 2. The Self and the Self-Image

So where does the idea of the "sort of person I am" come from? In short, the self-image is built moment by moment throughout life as a culmination of your interpretations of past experiences; successes and failures, triumphs and humiliations, and how you interpret others' reactions to these events. If you have told yourself countless times in the past that you WILL wake up early and take a brisk walk before work, or that you WILL take half of your meal home with you, and have failed to do so, you may begin to subconsciously and unknowingly accept these failures as "truths" about the sort of person you are. To make matters worse, you may even have gone to the extent of informing others of your intent; telling your husband of your intent to wake up early and walk before work. The next thing you know, you are hitting the snooze button instead of dragging yourself out of bed. Now, not only do you feel that you failed yourself, you are worried that your husband may be thinking less of you as well. Over time, these deductions that we make about ourselves imprint on our subconscious, making us "the sort of people we are."

Imprinting the Self-Image

Let's expand on this idea of imprinting ideas on the self-image. We now know that our self-image is subject to the imprinting of ideas through our exposure to past experiences. But do all past experiences affect us in the same way? According to Maltz, there are three factors that vary the degree at which our self-image is affected by past events; (1) Authoritative Source, (2) Intensity, and (3) Repetition.

Authoritative Source refers to our interpretation of the validity of someone else's reaction to an event in our past. For example, let's say you are at the onset of your latest weight loss attempt. Extremely excited, you rush home to tell your husband you have just signed up for a VIP All-Inclusive Membership to a local health club. Expecting to be greeted with praise of your newly found motivation, you are crushed when ambushed with "That's fine, but you have a perfectly good treadmill downstairs that you don't use." If your husband is an authoritative source in your life, you might take this to heart, allowing the idea that you will not utilize the membership to resonate. "After all, he does know me pretty well. I guess I'll cancel the membership."

Intensity, the next component of imprinting, refers to just how strongly we interpret someone else's reaction to be. Take our previous example, except this time, your husband retorts "What the hell did you do that for? You wasted thousands of dollars of on that treadmill downstairs and all it does is collect dust! More money down the drain!" In this instance, the strength and intensity of your husband's reaction may leave a larger imprint on your self-image.

Repetition, the final component of imprinting, is fairly self-explanatory. Again let's visit the above example. Somehow you find the will to "prove him wrong", going to the health club every day. And every day you are confronted with statements such as "You don't have to prove anything to me. Just go ahead and cancel the membership." Hearing these statements over and over can create a stronger imprint on the self-image.

Willpower is a Fickle Friend

A known fact that has been well established, once these "truths" have been imprinted, it is unfeasible for you to act differently for any length of time. Although brave attempts may be made through the exertion of willpower, and brief exodus from the self-image may be realized, you will soon experience what Maltz called the "Snap-Back" effect. Contemplate the person who joins the gym and goes religiously every day for the first month or so of the New Year. Better yet, contemplate the person who makes it their mission to lose weight, and does so through willpower alone, only to regain it. It is in this theory that I found my first parallel idea with Maltz. I have a saying that I often use with my clients,

> *"Willpower is a fickle friend. By your side when times are good. Nowhere to be found when times are bad."*

If we are destined to act out as our self-image dictates, and willpower has no long-lasting effect, then what are we to do? After all, our self-image is a construct of past experiences. Are we doomed to experience life as dictated by past events, fruitlessly attempting to "will" ourselves to a thinner self, a healthier self, a better self? I think you already know the answer to that loaded question. Of course not. If we continue to think of the self-image as an invisible force field of limitation, any goal we set that exists outside of that self-image will be unattainable, or unmaintainable. Yet, we continually set external goals of self-improvement because we do not see the invisible self-image, standing directly in our path, laughing at our futile attempts of willpower. The answer lies in focusing on internal goals; goals that exist within our belief that they are able to be accomplished. Therefore, with each accomplishment of these smaller goals, we experience a strengthening and expanding of the self-image, allowing for future goals to be set larger and larger. It is here that we begin to realize our true potential, as seen in Figure 3. Self-Image Expansion.

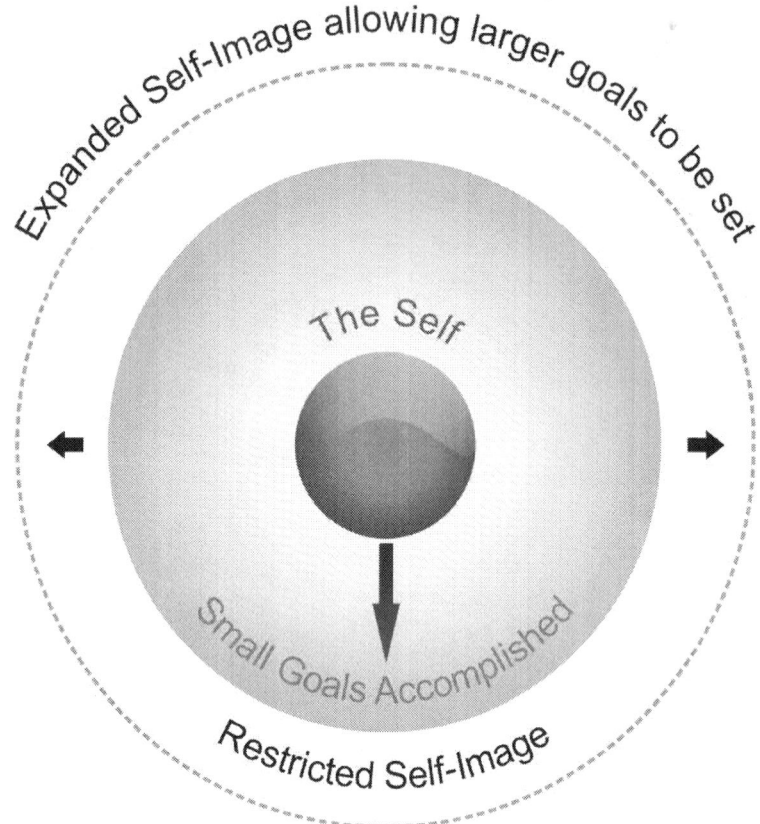

Figure 3. Self-Image Expansion

Your Subconscious Machine

In applying a scientific approach to the inner working of the mind, Dr. Maltz explained that the title "subconscious mind" is misleading. He writes, "…the so-called 'subconscious mind' is not a mind at all, but a goal-striving servo-mechanism consisting of the brain and nervous system which is used and directed by the mind." Maltz also interchangeably used the terms servo-mechanism and creative mechanism. More important than what you choose to call it, the servo-mechanism is much like a computer that exists in the subconscious mind. In this day and age, we all know how wonderful a computer can be at making our lives simpler, completing vast amounts of work in fractions of a second; the same task requiring our conscious minds more than a lifetime to complete.

It may seem simplistic in nature to assume that we can solely tell our subconscious mind to complete a task, such as weight loss, and it will do so accordingly. However, here is proof that we utilize this servo-mechanism countless times each day. Maltz is renowned for stating "If you can remember, worry, or tie your shoe, you can succeed with Psycho-Cybernetics." Every morning you wake up and go through the same routine. Do you consciously think about brushing your teeth? Sure, you might consciously think to yourself that you are about to engage in that task, but do you consciously say to yourself "pick up the brush, place toothpaste on the brush head, place the brush into the mouth, move your hand back and forth while holding the brush handle, making sure to thoroughly cleanse every tooth?" In another example, how many times have you consciously thought about your route on your drive to work? Yes, the conscious mind must be available to deal with street signals, pedestrians, etc. But each of us has thought to ourselves, "I don't even remember the drive today." These are very simple examples of the servo-mechanism at work.

The goal was programmed, and the proper result was achieved.

It is of utmost importance for us to remember just what the limitations of a computer are. For example, take that same computer that's in your home or on your desk at work that is completing countless tasks for you every day. That physical computer becomes far less valuable without the programming that it contains. In short, the hardware is useless without the software. Imagine that computer now has a virus, in other words, a disruption in its programming. Is that computer going to effectively solve the tasks that you assign to it?

So, each and every one of us is granted at birth this marvelous internal computer, or servo-mechanism, that lies in our subconscious; a goal-striving mechanism with a sole purpose of achieving whatever it is you tell it to do...WHATEVER IT IS YOU TELL IT TO DO. The servo-mechanism is completely objective and impersonal. It has no "prepackaged programming" of sorts, other than the instinctual programming to survive. You are the programmer of your servo-mechanism. If you provide it with goals of success, success shall be reaped. Should you program it with goals of failure, even inadvertently, such results will be provided. At this point I am sure you are questioning this statement. After all, at the onset of every attempt to lose weight, you do not tell your servo-mechanism that you want to fail. True enough. However, we must revisit the self-image for a moment; that invisible force field that acts as a filter between our conscious thought and our subconscious servo-mechanism. If you try to consciously communicate a goal of weight loss to your subconscious servo-mechanism, it must first pass through the self-image filter. If that success goal of weight loss is not consistent with your current self-image, meaning that you either consciously or subconsciously do not believe you are able to accomplish that goal, it will be rejected. Think of it like this. With a negative self-image, you have metaphorically installed an anti-success program on your internal servo-mechanism, much like an antivirus protection program on the computer in your office. Accept in this situation, malicious programs are not being blocked, but your goals of success are, as you can see in Figure 4. Self-Image Filter.

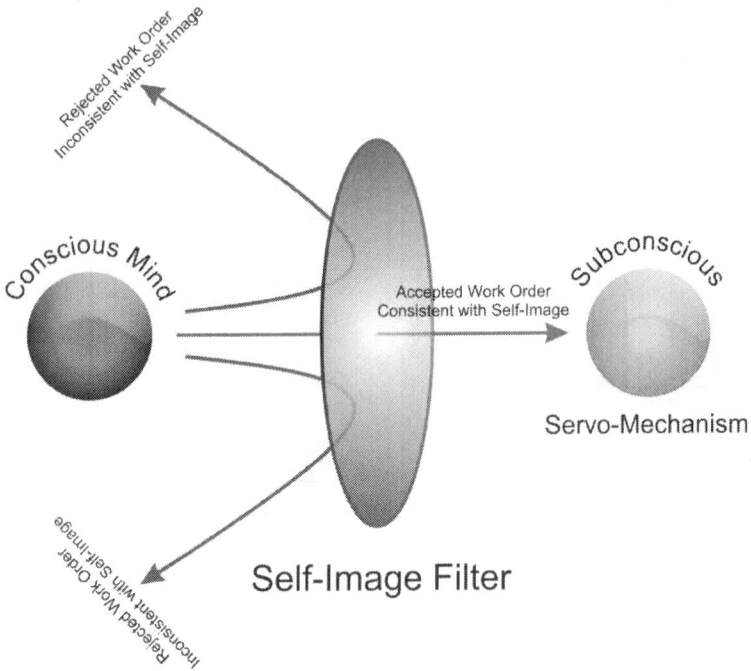

Figure 4. Self-Image Filter

This again reiterates why attempting to set external goals that are outside of our force field, or that are inconsistent with the self-image, will result in failure. Again, true success can only be realized when the self-image is strengthened and grown. Only at that time can goals of successful weight loss be effectively communicated to your subconscious servo-mechanism, which will then, if practiced repetitiously, begin to adopt these new healthy behaviors as habit. However, if the self-image is governed by previous imprinting of negative, or failure ideas, we must first change those imprints through a formula including "learning, practicing, and experiencing new habits of thinking, imagining, remembering, and acting in order to" (1) develop of an adequate and realistic self-image, and (2) use your servo-mechanism to generate successful weight loss effortlessly.

What About Genetics?

By this point, you might have very well contemplated the idea of genetic predisposition and one' ability (or inability) to lose weight. I don't blame you. In today's media, you are bombarded with research suggesting that your genes and hormones may have much to do with how your body will deal with excess fat. It is only then logical to think that in our genetic code is written our destiny on the scale, wrapped with a pretty little double-helix bow. However, I cannot believe that to be the case. Let me pose this example to you. It is well accepted that coming from a family history of alcoholism strongly correlates to a genetic predisposition for future alcoholics in that family's lineage. Does this mean it is futile to fight it? What if that person never has a drink in their life? Are they still destined to be an alcoholic? I do understand that there is a difference, mainly, that one cannot simply abstain from food, as a recovering alcoholic might abstain from alcohol. However, accepting for one moment that you are genetically predetermined to be unable to achieve your weight loss goals is absolutely intolerable. As Maltz would put it, "an excuse of the saddest kind."

Getting Started

As this Chapter comes to a close, I have laid the platform on which we build the realization of your weight loss goals, and will leave you with the following thought. We agree that the self-image governs our goal-striving machine, the self-image. Additionally, it is safe to say that at some point in your life, your self-image has been negatively imprinted through an authoritative source, with intensity, and repetitiously.

So here is your first step towards Zero Resistance Weight Loss. If you are reading this book, you more than likely have accepted me as an authoritative source. After all, I am a nutrition professional who himself has lost well over one hundred pounds. Well then, *I* am personally telling you with *GREAT INTENSITY*, that your weight loss goals are not only achievable, but have been right under your nose this whole time. The last part of the imprinting equation is up to you; repetition. Throughout the Chapters in this book, you will be exposed to concepts and examples intended to illustrate how you can put these theories into practice, helping you to achieve you weight loss goals. This book was not intended to be read passively. You can impose the final component of imprinting, repetition, by actively engaging in these activities. It's up to you.

Chapter Two

A Path to Success

As discussed in the previous Chapter, we have demonstrated that each and every one of us has three unique components, all of which play an irreplaceable role in ultimately deciding what results as our successes and failures, including our journey to lose weight; (1) the conscious mind, (2) the self-image, and (3) the subconscious servo-mechanism.

Is It My Imagination...?

In simplistic terms, the conscious mind is responsible for offering ideas and commands; the programming, if you will. This process might begin as a humble thought. That thought can then grow with the use of Creative Imagination. We have just added this fourth component to the formula, as can be seen in Figure 5. The Formula.

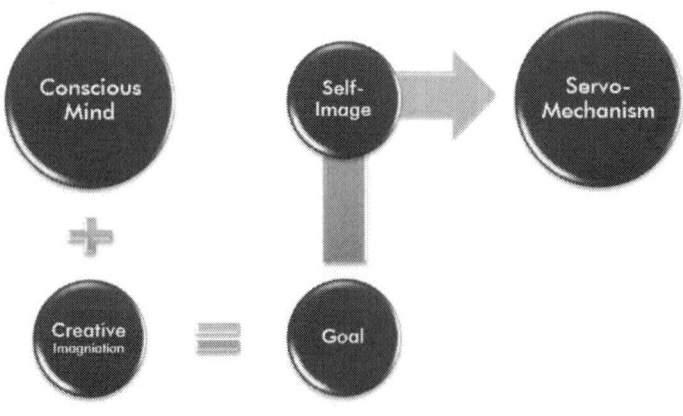

Figure 5. The Formula

For example, an idea pops into your head one day, "I have got to shed a few of these extra pounds." At this point, it is pretty much just an inoperable thought. However, if you engage your creative imagination while stirring in this thought, you can begin to envision the process that needs to unfold. You see yourself going to the grocery store after work to pick up some fresh fruit and vegetables. You see yourself starting your health club membership tomorrow. What I am actually describing here is the use of your creative imagination to help define the command. This command is now ready to be shuttled over to the subconscious servo-mechanism for completion. The subconscious servo-mechanism would be the processor of this equation. Similar to a computer, the programmer (the conscious mind) issues a command, and can then rely on the servo-mechanism to handle the task. The self-image acts as the filter between the programming commands from the conscious mind to the subconscious servo-mechanism. Remember our analogy, as represented in Figure 6. Inconsistent Programming. The self-image will act as "virus-protection" between the conscious and subconscious minds. The only difference is the self-image is not protecting your subconscious from malicious software. Rather, it will only allow ideas and commands to filter through if they are consistent with your current paradigm of beliefs, system of ideas, or the sort of person you are.

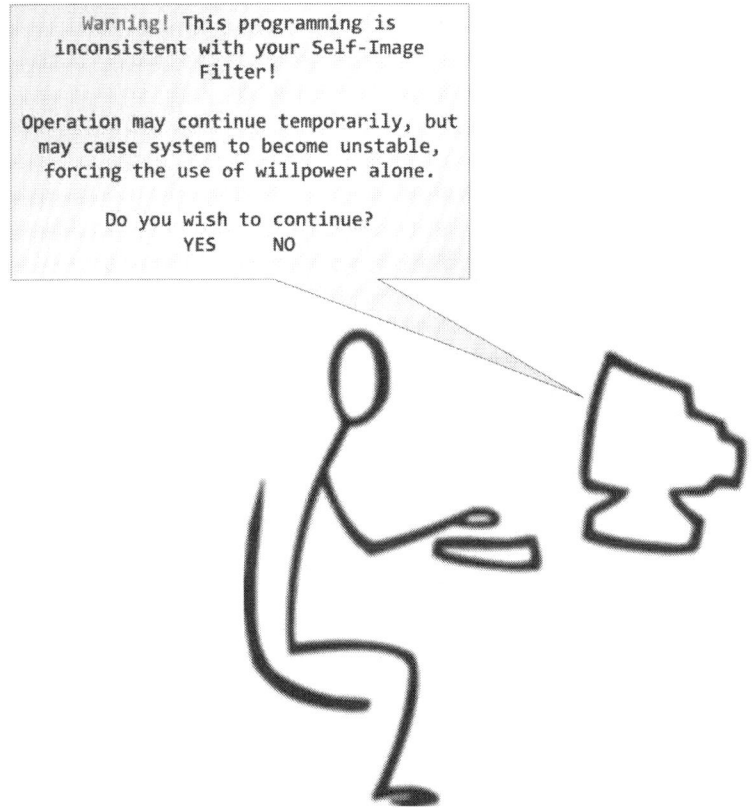

Figure 6. Inconsistent Programming

It is important to remember that the subconscious servomechanism is a completely impartial and impersonal mechanism. It does not natively contain a morality indicator. Nor will it judge what you ask it to do. Those tasks lie within the self-image. If you are someone who has experienced years of countless failed attempts at weight loss, chances are you have constructed a negative filter within the self-image of being someone who is unable to lose weight. That is not to say you do not consciously attempt to lose weight. Simply put, since your self-image filter blocks those commands to the servo-mechanism, you are left to attempt to lose weight with only the aid of sheer willpower and effort, as these exist in the conscious mind. The solution is found in reprogramming the self-image filter to allow success-type commands, while filtering out failure-type commands. Honestly, this process is not as difficult as you might think.

Navigating to Success

If you continue to think of this process as a machine in action, it might be more easily explained if I rephrase like this. The servo-mechanism has a built in navigation system, or GPS, similar to a car. Like any computer, your internal GPS programming might malfunction. You put in your desired destination of weight loss. However, if the self-image reflects that of a negative outlook, your internal GPS will continue to guide you towards failure-type outcomes. You may very well consciously know which direction you want to go. However, your GPS keeps telling you to go in the other direction. You know you want to make it to the gym, but your GPS keeps telling you to go home. You know you want to pick up some healthy food from the store, but your GPS keeps telling you to pick up a pizza.

I remind you of the example from the previous Chapter regarding your spouse scorning you for purchasing a health club membership. In this example, you were taken down a path that led to your self-image bowing the authoritative, intense, and repetitive nature of their negative remarks. At this point your self-image was filtering out, or rejecting, all positive commands stemming from the conscious mind. You began down that spiral decent of discouragement, doubting your capabilities to succeed, ultimately leading to your conscious disregard for your goal, weight loss. Your servo-mechanism became your automatic failure mechanism, acting as a guidance system to failure. Here is the good news. It is only logical that we deduce from this example that if the servo-mechanism can have a predetermined destination of failure, you can change the destination by engaging the Automatic Success Mechanism.

The Success Mechanism in Action

Here is a basic introduction to how to properly utilize your servo-mechanism. First, you must choose your target, or goal. I will use travel as an example. I live in Youngstown, Ohio, directly in the middle of, and about 60 miles from Pittsburgh and Cleveland. I am on my way to an Indians game, so I set my target, or goal, to arrive in Cleveland.

The second step is to engage in action. While I have consciously set my goal, that won't get me very far. At this point, I can use my creative imagination to determine my best possible route. I decide that the turnpike is a good idea, since I can drive a little bit faster. I get into my car, and away I go. At this point, I am barely using my conscious mind, as I have been driving for years, and have driven this route so many times in the past. My servo-mechanism is engaged.

The third step is critical; Continual Course Correction. It would be a wonderful world if no unforeseen obstacles ever jumped into our path en route towards our goal. Sadly enough, this is not the case. As I drive along, a deer abruptly crosses my path. I have dealt with this before. Without even thinking, I press the brake and switch lanes. Not much of big deal. I have learned how to deal with that situation in the past and my brain remembered it. A few miles down the road, traffic comes to complete standstill. As it is important to me to get to the game on time, I course correct, in the most literal sense of the term, choosing to take the next exit to see if I can find a faster way to get there. As I look for landmarks to redirect me to my target, my "low gas" indicator light comes on. I swing into a gas station and fill up, and actually take the time to ask for directions. Just a little over an hour after leaving my driveway, I get to the stadium, just in time to see the first pitch. Goal accomplished!

The last part of this example details what makes this third step so crucial. My course correction must be continual until the goal is met. At no time did I say "Oh no. A deer is in the road. Better not go any further." Nor did I say "Out of gas. Better stay here forever" or "Traffic jam. Might as well pull over."

Through continual course correction I was able to meet my goal, arriving in Cleveland. This is an example of one of two general types of servo-mechanisms. This first type is when the target, or goal, is known to exist. I have been to Cleveland countless times. I know that it exists about 60 miles northwest of Youngstown. The second type of servo-mechanism action is engaged when the target is unknown, and the objective becomes to locate that target, or goal. There were examples of this during my drive to Cleveland. I hoped that there was an alternate route when I got off the turnpike during the traffic jam. I hoped there was a gas station when my indicator came on. The pivotal word is "hoped". This can be replaced with the word "believed". My goal would not have been achieved if I had not hoped or believed that there was an alternate route, or a gas station nearby. Should I have believed that the turnpike was the sole route, or that the gas station by my home is the only one in existence, I would have probably given up on my goal pretty quickly. Here lies an absolutely fascinating attribute of the human brain. Not only did I reach my goal through course correction, but my brain will remember the events that took place, store the information, so that my servo-mechanism may draw upon it in future events. Maybe next time I will not take the turnpike at five o'clock, as I know that traffic can get backed up. Although I hope to never need to, I now know a place that I can conveniently get gas, as well as take an alternate route if necessary. Additionally, my course corrections were quick, and decisive. The more frequently we experience similar events, the faster we can expedite decisive conclusions, to the point where it becomes habit. Habits exist in the servo-mechanism, as no effort is needed to act out of habit.

A Tale of Weight Loss Success

I have illustrated the use of the servo-mechanism through a rather arbitrary example of driving to Cleveland. Let's take a look at how this process might apply to weight loss. To start, you must first choose your goal, or target. This might be a specific weight, or a more unspecific goal of weight loss in general (we will discuss effective goal and objective setting in the chapters to come). Our first step is accomplished and you have set your goal to lose 25 lbs. Is this goal of known or unknown origin? It can be quite discouraging to strive for a goal if you do not know if it exists. Have you ever lost 25 lbs.? If not, you might deduce that this is an unknown goal. I will challenge you to think differently here. It is scientific fact that if your caloric intake is less than that of your caloric expenditure, your body will utilize fuel that has been stored as body fat, and weight loss will occur. Is this overly simplistic? Yes. But true, nonetheless. Therefore, I would encourage you to believe that your goal in fact DOES EXIST!

On to the second step; taking action. A goal is of no use without this second step. So you've decided to implement strategies that you have used in the past, heard via the media, or through an appointment with a Registered Dietitian or your physician.

> ...You begin eating breakfast every morning.

> ...You begin packing your lunch for work, along with a mid-morning and mid-afternoon snack.

> ...You stock your refrigerator and pantry with whole grains, lean proteins, fruits, and vegetables.

> ...You enlist your neighbor to begin taking after-dinner walks.

In essence, you are drawing upon information that has been stored in your brain, learned from past experiences in your attempts to lose weight. Maybe they have worked in the past; maybe they haven't. Maybe you have never even used them before. But for whatever reason, you have decided to implement these strategies, or take action, to reach your goal.

Next is that ever-critical third step; continual course correction. Along your path towards your weight loss goal, you inadvertently hit your snooze button one morning, making it impossible to make time for breakfast. As a result, you put it on your to-do list to stop at the store to pick up a box of breakfast bars to keep at work so this situation doesn't pop up again. Course corrected. Upon arriving at work, you realize you have forgotten to pack your lunch. No problem, as you decide you can drive to the local fast food restaurant and choose to order a salad with chicken breast. Course corrected. Next, you get home for dinner only to realize your ravenous teenage sons have eaten just about everything that you planned on making for your inaugural "healthy family" dinner. But you are determined not to let this discourage you. You rummage through your kitchen finding just enough to make a quick dinner that fits into your plan. Course corrected. As if your day hasn't been bad enough, your neighbor calls to inform you that she is feeling under the weather and will be unable to walk with you for a couple of days. Okay, time to make a new playlist on your iPod® and take matters into your own hands. It's not quite as entertaining as a pleasant conversation with your neighbor, but taking a walk by yourself will do. Course corrected!

If I were to continue on with this example, I am sure that the length of this book would rapidly increase; and a great many readers would never make it Chapter Three. There are several instances of course correction in this story which illustrate the *Automatic Success Mechanism* in action. With every obstacle, a quick and decisive evaluation of the situation was made, then choosing the most effective and efficient decision that was consistent with reaching the goal. If the automatic failure mechanism was in gear, responses may have resembled something more like, "I'll just eat a doughnut at work for breakfast", "I'll get a candy bar out of the vending machine for lunch, "Looks like we'll be ordering a pizza for dinner", and "I'll start walking as soon as the neighbor feels better; maybe next Monday."

Procrastination – The Bain of Success

That last statement brings me to the next point. Ponder the previous statement for a moment. *"I'll start...as soon as..."* Does that sound familiar? It does to me. I couldn't even begin to tell you how many times I have muttered that statement in my head. *"I'll start...*

...exercising as soon as I get off these first few pounds."

...watching my diet after the holidays."

...on Monday."

...the first of the month."

...January 1st."

The list could go on and on. I am assuming that if you are reading this book, there has been some point in your life that you have attempted to lose weight. More than likely there have been several times that you have attempted to lose weight. But if we look at it more rationally, the goal of weight loss was set that very first time, and hasn't gone anywhere since. It might have sat dormant from time to time, but it was still there, eating away at you from the inside out. So what can we deduce from this? We can deduce that your goal has never changed; you simply did not correctly utilize your servo-mechanism, leaving out that critical third step of continual course correction. At very best, you did not engage in such course correction in a quick and decisive manner. You corrected your course, but it may have been several months or years in between. The purpose of continual course correction, the exact process that your automatic success mechanism is designed for, is to make corrections to get back on course as soon as possible, in the most effective and efficient manner possible. So why is it that we choose to act otherwise, and how might we change that?

Fuel Your Fire

While this book contributes how to apply the science of Psycho-Cybernetics and the works of Dr. Maxwell Maltz to weight loss, there is another icon in this field that we may harvest priceless advice. Napolean Hill is a pioneer in deciphering the characteristics of people who achieve paramount success. In his classic work Think and Grow Rich, Hill details thirteen characteristics shared by the wealthiest and most successful people of his generation. While he concentrated his research on the gathering of wealth, many of the same principles apply to a more broad sense of success. Two of these characteristics apply here; *Desire and Persistence.* Before the process of taking action towards achieving any goal can be engaged, an unbridled desire for achieving that goal must be developed. This desire must be cultivated to the point of eruption, where there is absolutely no other option other than moving towards that goal. But as you well know, even the hottest fire and highest flames extinguish over time if not given adequate fuel. So enters persistence. Just as desire built the fire, persistence is the fuel that keeps that fire burning strong. Without persistence, procrastination steps in, acting as the bucket of water that can extinguish even the deepest of desires.

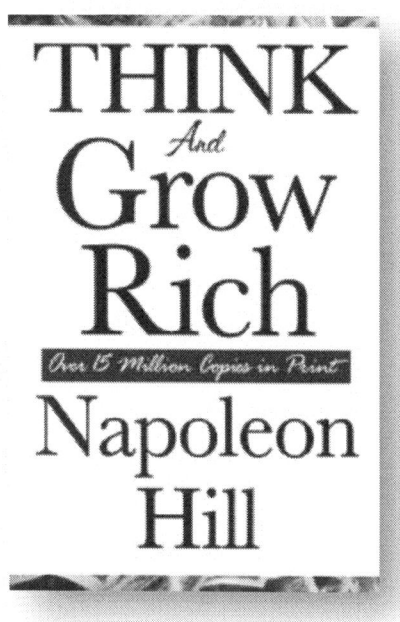

Figure 7. THINK AND GROW RICH, Napolean Hill

My question for you is this. If you have set your goal to lose weight at some point in your past, what is stopping you? It is unquestionably so that obstacles will always be in your path. That is why you were gifted with your servo-mechanism; to course correct. Maybe your previous attempts have left you without positive results. But I would challenge that statement by saying the only feedback that is guaranteed in life is negative feedback. We learn from doing things the wrong way, not the right way. The more we fail, the more lessons we can learn about what doesn't work, taking us closer and closer to what does work. Reminisce on your failed attempts, and take from them only the lesson that was taught. After that, discard it like an apple core that has been eaten clean of all valuable nutrients. If you are honest with yourself, we can agree on this next statement. At some point, you will again attempt to lose weight. That goal has been branded into your mind long ago. Stoke that fire we call desire until it is white hot, and move into action. And when that fire begins to fade, throw persistence at it like kindle and logs. The mistakes will continue. Learn from them, course correct, and achieve your goal. It is your destiny, and what your servo-mechanism was built to do. I have a saying that I often use with my clients for just such an occasion.

"I envy the person with countless failures, and pity the person with just one."

Chapter Three

It's All in Your Head

In the previous Chapter, I unveiled the fourth component of the formula which can switch your servo-mechanism into success-gear, transforming it into the automatic success mechanism that it was designed to be. This component is creative imagination. Our creative imagination is the portal to the construction of a true perception of ourselves. Believe it or not, this perception will undeniably be accepted as true, whether immediately or over time. Thinking in this regard, if you effectively present an idea to your imagination, then employing your imagination to create a picture that is so vividly true that you have no choice but to begin to accept this as reality, then this is not far from the idea of hypnosis.

Hypnotized

The concept of hypnosis often summons two strong, and equally opposite opinions of the matter. On one hand, you have your group of people who believe whole-heartedly that hypnosis, suggestion, and mental imagery can be effectively used to create such a strong perception in the mind, that when under hypnosis, one will act "as-if" the presented idea were actually true. One the other hand, you have your group of naysayers. This would be your group of people who would chalk hypnosis up to being nothing more than a parlor trick, used by magicians and the like. Regardless of which group you find yourself in, there is a wealth of research that has produced results supporting that the use of mental imagery and hypnosis, and if presented correctly, can yield a psychosomatic response. That is to say, if the person experiencing the mental imaging creates a vivid enough picture, the body will automatically generate a physiologic response.

Unfortunately, hypnosis tends to be associated with common pictures of the man on stage being convinced that he is a dog, barking and scratching his ear with his hind leg. A more credible framework must be developed for me to expect you to believe that your mind contains this type of power. In the September 2007 issue of the Journal of Psychosomatic Research, researcher Peter Whorwell investigated the efficacy of hypnosis on reducing the symptoms associated with irritable bowel syndrome. For those of you who are not familiar with this condition, irritable bowel syndrome is not well understood, however, it is known that symptoms include paralyzing nausea, back aches, and urologic and gynecologic pain, to name a few. While admittedly not understanding the mechanism behind the relief, Whorwell explains that "it (hypnosis) can modulate gastrointestinal physiology, alter the central processing of noxious stimuli, and even influence immune function." In layman's terms, this simply means that Whorwell found evidence that hypnosis can reduce the nauseating side effects of irritable bowel, as well as stimulate an immune response. In another instance, chronicled in the May 2011 issue of the International Journal of Adolescent Medicine and Health, researchers determined in an experiment including thirty three children, that thirty of the participants were able to voluntarily increase their peripheral skin temperature through mental imagery and suggestion.

To be clear, I am not suggesting that I can hypnotize you into losing weight. That is not the intent of this book. Additionally, I do not wish to clutter these pages with statistical analysis and support. I simply wish to present the possibility of the power of the psychological over the physiological, and I will leave my assessment with one additional real-world example. Take someone who battles anorexia. We have all seen the dramatic daytime talk shows displaying a young girl or boy undeniably self-convinced that they are overweight, despite the rigid bones protruding from under their skin, and the dangerously low double digit weight that stares back at them when standing on the scale. Isn't this simply another example of hypnosis? This situation includes an idea, or suggestion, that has been built into the imagination of the anorectic for years, fabricating a perception of "truth", to such an extent that the physiologic response is that of self-imposed starvation. I think it would be fair to say that an anorectic is living in a hypnotic state.

Given the facts presented, is it reasonable to assume that each and every one of us has the capability of being hypnotized on some level, no matter how minor, unnoticeable, or unrecognizable? Or even possibly that we already are living in a hypnotic state? Maltz would say yes, and that this hypnotic state is governed by the self-image. Here is his example of situation where one's perception of the event yielded an unnecessary result.

> *The human brain and nervous system are engineered to react automatically and appropriately to problems and challenges in the environment. For example, a man does not need to stop and think that self-survival requires that he run if he meets a grizzly bear on a trail. He does not need to decide to become afraid. The fear response is both automatic and appropriate. First, it makes him want to flee. The fear that triggers bodily mechanisms that "soup up" his muscles so that he can run faster than he has ever run before. His heart beat is quickened. Adrenaline, a powerful muscle stimulant, is poured into the bloodstream. All bodily functions not necessary to running are shut down. The stomach stops working and all available blood is sent to the muscles. Breathing is much faster and the oxygen supply to the muscles is increased manyfold.*

This is undoubtedly an appropriate physiologic response. The situation produced the formation of an idea by the man confronted by the bear, which led to an emotional and physiologic response. However, what if the man were to learn that this "bear" was nothing more than a friend in a bear costume playing a trick on him. Is the response still appropriate? Should someone be that afraid of their friend? This example just goes to show you that our reaction to a situation is less based in reality, and more so based on our perception of reality.

Here is another example more in tune with the topic of weight loss. Two friends, Mary and Sue, set out to lose weight. Both join the local health club and employ the services of personal trainers for assistance with their exercise routine. Unknown to the two ladies, Mary gets the luck of the draw, acquiring the assistance of a seasoned professional. Meanwhile, Sue procures the assistance of the trainer still slightly wet behind the ears. Although her progress is slow, Mary is showered with praise for her accomplishments, and positive encouragement to continue with persistence. Sue, on the other hand, is met with negative response to her slow progress. "You need to stop being so lazy. You'll never lose a single pound at this rate", her trainer scolds. Both of these women have the same goal, or target; weight loss. Both are going through the same exact exercise regimen, and both are following the same diet plan. Mary has the benefit of external sources helping her to create a perception that she can accomplish her goal. Sue has the hindrance of external sources creating a perception of hopelessness. Who do you think will succeed? To be more concise, who do you believe will be persistent, correct their mistakes, and continue striving towards their goal?

The reaches of living in a fabricated hypnotic state, that is, one of false perception, far outreach those explained in these examples. How many of us continually and effortlessly believe that we have no control over what the scale should read when we step on it in the morning? How did you come to such conclusions? Through the formation of your self-image via your perception of personal historical events, that's how. Through what you imagined the case to be, and just how strongly you imagined it to be so. How many times have you experienced a failure in your journey in weight loss? I have experienced many. Did I allow that failure to manifest itself as the "truth", that I am a weight loss failure? Maybe at one point in my life, but not anymore.

Dehypnotizing Yourself

The pieces of the puzzle are all laid out for you here on these pages. How will you effectively change your self-image to create a new and true perception of reality, that you can lose weight? It is a three-step process.

1. You must first identify any false conceptions you hold regarding your inability to lose weight.
2. You must then challenge these false conceptions, allowing your conscious, and subsequently your subconscious mind, that this perception is nothing more than illusion.

3. You must then replace these false conceptions with perceptions of success.

Mental Practice Makes Perfect

To recap this elaboration of the power of mental imaging, when such a vivid mental picture is created, the body has no choice but to yield an emotional and physiologic response that would mimic that of the situation were actually happening around you. To be more specific, your central nervous system absolutely cannot distinguish between actual, physical experience and that of vivid imagination. Taking this fact a step further, we can feel confident that practicing something in our imagination can be just as beneficial as practicing in real life. This fact stands true for practicing a new skill, a sport, or simply acting out new traits that you wish to embody, such as those needed to achieve a healthy weight.

This notion is nothing new. Various professions use mental practice to improve on their skillset, with nothing in common between these professions other than that a certain skill is required to complete their task. In a classic example presented in *Psycho-Cybernetics*, Maltz cites *Research Quarterly's* testament to mental practice making perfect. In this experiment, a population of students was pretested for accuracy in shooting free throws in basketball. They were then broken down into three subgroups. The first group physically practiced shooting free throws for twenty days. The second group participated in no practice whatsoever.

The third group spent twenty minutes each day for the twenty days vividly imaging themselves practicing free throws. At the end of the twenty day experiment, each group was post-tested to determine the level of improvement. The first group, those who physically practiced, improved in accuracy by 24%. The second group, participating in no practice whatsoever, did not improve at all. The third group, engaging only in mental imaging practice, improved by 23%.

Mental imaging in sports is well-accepted as credible and downright necessary. From basketball, to golf, to baseball, and football alike; recreational, amateur, and professional athletes will attest to the benefit of mental imaging in accomplishing their goals. So you might not be an athlete, and are now wondering if this theory possibly doesn't apply to you. Outside of athletes, mental imaging has been effectively utilized in training surgeons, as well. In the March 2007 issue of the *Annals of Surgery*, surgeons demonstrated that, what they termed mental training, was actually more effective at increasing simulated surgical scores when calculated via checklist of procedures and tasks when compared to that of practical, traditional training. Again, you might not be a surgeon. But I pose this to you. In general, a specific skill set is required of both athletes and surgeons. As well, a specific skill set is required of those attempting to lose weight.

The idea of using mental imaging to rehearse the process of eating may sound silly, unproductive, and somewhat exhausting. To be honest, if you were to tell me this, I would probably agree with you. However, there is an infinite number of ways to utilize your imagination to create a perception of success. The essence of the benefit procured from success imaging is to be able to efficiently and effectively deliver a mental image of a desired outcome, or goal, to the servo-mechanism, allowing it to catapult you to the finish line. Before I expound on this idea, we must discuss a simple and organized way to put our imagination into action.

Just Picture It

In his works, Maltz coined the phrase "Theater of the Mind"; a rather fancy phrase for imagination. However, thinking in this mindset might help you to engage your creative mechanism, or imagination. It often helps to factor in ideas from past memories to initiate your mind's theater. Using these memories, we will construct an experience in your mind through a series of simple steps.

Step One – Choose Your Movie. First, you must decide on the movie that you are about to watch. If I may, I would like to suggest a "feel good" flick; a story detailing your personal successes in weight loss.

Step Two – Infuse Reality. Let's inject some realistic illustrations from your memory. Imagine you are sitting in your favorite cinema auditorium. Remember the details from your previous trips, from the walk from your car, your walk through the lobby, etc. You enter the theater and choose your favorite seat. You look around, and there is no one else but you. You sink in to your seat, becoming more and more comfortable. The lights begin to dim, and the screen illuminates.

Step Three – Live Out the Movie. There you are, on the big screen, except, something is different. You know the person on screen is you, yet something is not the same, and that unfamiliarity is that you exude confidence. Although you are wearing your bathrobe, it is instantly noticeable that this version of you has something you have always yearned for; a slimmer body. This must be one of those movies where the end plays first and the subsequent events explain how the main character gets to that climactic occasion. You stand there in your bathroom; must have just gotten out of bed. You stand in front of the mirror, as you always do. Your robe slides off your shoulders and hits the floor. You can now see with more detail the personified efforts of fruitful hard work with exercise and healthy eating. Your body is more slender. Your arms and legs are toned. You take a few steps and take a deep breath and look down to see the scale in front of you. One more step up and the dial starts to move, bouncing back and forth. It seems like an eternity, and finally, the display reads your weight. Is this possible? It is the weight you have always wanted to see on that scale. The weight that has eluded you all of your life! Let's pause the movie for a moment.

Step Four – Make it Your Own. What emotions are you experiencing right now as you read this? Did you get a shiver running up your spine? If you did not experience a sensation of joy, that same feeling you get when you open the perfect birthday present, or when you open the door to find a delivery man presenting you a beautiful bouquet of flowers, I challenge you to go back through this script, this time with your eyes closed, letting your imagine fill in the creative gaps that my deficient creative writing skills leave out. Do not allow my shortcomings as a writer to ruin your experience. Make this sequence of events as elaborate as you see fit, making every detail your own. There are no limitations, as you are the writer, the director, and the producer of this epic story. Do not stop creating or elaborating until you produce that emotion felt only with that of the highest of successes. If you are having difficulties, let me provide you this piece of encouragement. This process gets much easier with practice. Recall from your memory the last movie you watched that evoked a positive emotion. Maybe a film whose main character was displayed as an underdog, standing up against terrible odds, only to achieve the inconceivable success. Do you remember the first time you saw *Rocky*? If a fictitious story can muster up emotions of that intensity, why shouldn't a story of your creation do the same?

The intention of this process is to yield what Maltz would call "that winning feeling", which we will discuss in depth in later chapters. For now, let it suffice that the purpose of evoking this emotion is simple. It creates an essence of success that will carry over into all of your actions throughout the day. If you evoke a strong enough emotion, it will literally be impossible for you to act differently than that emotion dictates. To be succinct, this emotion is motivational, which brings us to the next step in creating your mental movie.

Step Five – Rewind. Your movie started out in the end sequence, displaying the destination, building anticipation for you, the viewer, to understand the journey. It is your task to now go back and create a sequence of events in your mind's theater, just as detailed as the one that gave you "that winning feeling". Make a list of common obstacles and events that you face day in and day out that stand in your way of your weight loss goal. In your mind's theater, create a script for each of these situations detailing your actions that lead up to you conquering those situations. For example, I have personally encountered past failures in my attempt to exercise on a consecutive basis. However, I live by the saying "No one exercises to feel good during, but to feel good after." By being able to quickly engage my creative imagination, I can experience the feeling achieved after the activity. I can experience the feeling of accomplishment. I can experience the feeling of success. These experiences build drive and desire for the real thing, motivating me to get to the gym, or to hit the street for a quick run. After a while, this process becomes easier and easier. Eventually, this process becomes instantaneous. No longer do I have to build my motivation through a series of mental movies. Instead, my actions are that of habit, as my servo-mechanism has accepted the fact that my goal is health, and that exercise is part of my life.

By engaging your imagination to envision a version of yourself that is able to complete the tasks, and overcome the obstacles, eventually leading to your weight loss goal, your servo-mechanism will follow suit. You will find yourself living out your day, encountering real life situations that mimic those of your mental movies. This should create a "déjà vu effect", allowing your servo-mechanism to act out as you have practiced in your mind. Imagine you have difficulty maintaining your composure regarding portion size when you go out to eat. There you are, sitting at the table, contemplating if you have the willpower to not order an appetizer, order broccoli instead of French fries, or asking the server to spare you the temptation of a basket of bread. If you were to spend time playing out this sequence in your mind, you could experience the pride you might feel when you are able to do so. You might feel the satisfaction of choosing a well-balanced meal. Mentally experiencing these emotions over and over will create habit, making the decisions in real life situations all that more easy to handle. Additionally, willpower did not play a role. You were able to make these decisions merely because this is what you have practiced, and this is how you act. Simply put, it is "the type of person you are".

Chapter Four

Learning to Accept Reality

In the previous Chapter, we discussed the idea of creative mental imaging as a way to help enable the servo-mechanism engage in its main task; to strive for the goal that you've set. As strong as the creative imagination is, there is a negative influence holding you at bay. This invisible power is what we have referred to as the self-image; that force field, keeping you back from achieving those goals that exist just outside of it. We have even discussed the possibility that your self-image may be the result of living in a hypnotic state, blindly accepting the false truth that you are unable to achieve your weight loss goal. It is common sense that we now discuss how to remove these false truths and dehypnotize you, making the realization of your true potential not only a possibility, but a probability.

To revisit for a moment, hypnosis only occurs when one is convinced that the perception, or mental image, is so realistic, that the idea must be true. This can be completely true of those of us who at one time or another has thought that weight loss is an impossibility. In all of my experience in dealing with weight loss, both personally and professionally, I have never encountered someone who could not lose weight. The scientific proof exists all around us. If you are to lose weight, you must simply consume less calories than expended. However, we continually bombard ourselves with negative ideations regarding the difficulties of weight loss.

> *"I don't have time to exercise."*

> *"I haven't been able to stay on a diet for more than a month."*

> *"I can't control myself when I go out to eat."*

> *"The holidays unravel my best efforts."*

If you have ever recited any variation of one of these statements, it is very possible that you have hypnotized yourself into believing you can't lose weight. If you are ready to recognize that these limitations may be self-imposed, then you are ready to dehypnotize yourself.

Calling Your Bluff

The phrase "calling your bluff" originated from the game of poker. Its meaning consists of one player recognizing that another player may not have the good hand that they are acting like they have. Imagine you are playing poker and have what most would call a decent hand, maybe a low "three of a kind". Unbeknownst to you, your opponent has a weaker hand; only a pair of tens. By the rules of poker, you would win. However, your opponent decides to bet heavily in attempt to get you to fold your hand. Your opponent is playing a bluff. If you believe this false truth, that his hand is better than yours, you will fold, accepting that you "can't" beat his hand. After all, your opponent is considered the best poker player of your friends, always takes home the biggest pot, and is acting quite confidently of his chances of winning (a representation of authority, repetition, and intensity). But this time you decide you're going to "pay to see" the cards, and call the bet. You have just called the bluff, and the rewards will be great.

If you have acknowledged that your self-image may be the result of a few false truths about your inability to lose weight accepted along your life's journey, you have been folding your winning hand. It is important to realize that the hand you're dealt is the hand you're dealt, but how you play it makes all the difference. Right now, your self-image is your opponent. Through repetitious past experiences being unable to successfully lose weight, you have created a self-image that makes you feel that you cannot win. As soon as you realize that your self-image is bluffing, the pot is yours for the taking. By challenging each and every limitation that your self-image is imposing on you, you will be able to push the borders of the self-image out, making way for successful completion of your goals.

Keeping in line with the poker analogy, it is important to realize that at no time has your hand of cards (your potential ability) changed. You have possessed that same hand this whole time. It is when you recognize that your hand is strong enough to beat your self-imposed limitations that you will expand your self-image.

False Measures; a Common Thief

A valuable message can be conveyed from a very brief history lesson. Many centuries ago, people often used parts of their body to measure things. For example, the term "foot" was introduced as a simple way to express an estimated amount of distance. This gave the ability for anyone with a foot to simply walk off, in a heel-to-toe manner, the distance between two points. Of course, the variations of human foot size can be large. This may have become a problem with early merchants selling goods by length, such as fabric. Obviously, if you were buying a foot of expressive fabric such as silk, you would probably want to find a merchant with the largest feet. Subsequently, the need for standardization of units of length, weight, volume, etc., proceeded to give us the finite and precise measurements we have today become accustom to, lest we painfully learn the lesson, "not by another man's foot".

With this in mind, your foot is your foot, and you are you. Yet we continually compare ourselves to others. This is a prime example of false measurement. The primary lesson to be learned in the pages of this book is to realize the unutilized potential of the self, not someone else. Your comparisons should stem from within. Compare the present version of yourself to the past version of yourself. Are you progressing? Compare the present version of yourself to the one that lies just outside your self-image.

"Now" and "Then"

One of my frequented exercise routines is running. Now let me be clear. What I call "running" includes a duration of time where my efforts range from briskly walking to slow jogging, then increasing my speed to that of ranging between a fast jog to slow run. Over time, I have improved on my capabilities to "run" more than I "walk". Some might refer to this as interval running. Others might say it is the lack of ability to run consistently at a fast pace. So I will pose the question, am I a good runner? Not if I were to compare myself to Usain Bolt, the Jamaican World and Olympic record holder in 100 meter sprint. And what if I were to then compare Usain Bolt to Geoffrey Mutai of Kenya, who in 2011 ran the fastest ever Boston Marathon, at two hours, three minutes, and two seconds? Would this comparison matter to either of them? Probably not, and this is the reason. Each of us has one thing is common. We are all striving towards a goal. Geoffrey Mutai may have set out to run the Boston Marathon faster than anyone has before, but he undoubtedly started that race trying to beat his own personal best time. Usain Bolt may have set out to be the world's fastest sprinter, and he accomplished that. And with every race, I am confident that he attempts to break that record time that he has set. I have no drive or desire to be that of a record holding runner, and if I were to compare myself to either of these individuals, I would probably find myself to be quite discouraged. My drive and desire was formed by my goal of first, weight loss, and then, weight maintenance. Running was simply a tool for me to achieve my goal. I do take pride in the fact that, when I consistently make it to the treadmill, I increase my ability to run greater distances at higher speeds for longer durations of time. This pride is derived not from being faster than the person next to me, but by being better than the "me of yesterday". As Maltz so eloquently put it,

> *It is not the knowledge of actual inferiority in skill or knowledge that gives us an inferiority complex and interferes with our living. It is the feeling of inferiority that does this.*

It does not matter that you cannot walk as fast, or as long as the person on the treadmill next to you at the gym. What matters is that you are there pushing yourself to be better than you were yesterday. It doesn't matter that you are not able to maintain the strictest of diets. What matters is that you are attempting to improve your diet at all. Lastly, it doesn't matter that you don't fit into the size small clothing worn by the catalog models, or by your friends. What matters is that your size double extra-large clothes have made their way to the Salvation Army because you are now wearing a single extra-large.

In reality, we are all inferior to others in some ways, and superior to others in different respects. There is a high probability that I am currently better than you in regards to being able to lose weight and keep it off. There would be little probability of you reading this book if that was not the case. I achieve no sense of pride in making that assumption, as I understand the fact that you are undoubtedly superior to me in many other skill sets. If anything, I achieve a sense of duty in assisting each and every reader of this book in realizing that my comparing myself to you is unproductive. Comparison of "myself now" to "myself then" is motivating. Comparison of my current self to who I envision that I can become is priceless. All of this is because I use the same method of measure, which is me.

Superior Failures

Of course, there are those people in the world who walk with arrogance, seldom showing regard for others. This is commonly referred to as a "superiority complex." Many experts would tell you that there is no such thing, and would go on to explain that the superiority expressed through these people's actions is simply overcompensation for their shortcomings. While their actions may be inexcusable, and maybe even hurtful, once you realize that this is an expression of their own inner demons, their actions should become fairly arbitrary to you.

Then there are those who I refer to as the "anti-superiors", or "success vampires". These people can be the most damaging to your weight loss goals. I often hear stories from my clients that have a similar core. They all involve these anti-superior people. What makes them so dangerous is their innate ability, whether conscious or not, to remove any motivation that you currently possess. Signs of anti-superior people might be those who tell you:

> *"Just split dessert with me. You deserve it!"*

> *"You've exercised enough this week. You can skip today and go shopping with me."*

These are people who find security in, not only residing in their own inferiority, but in creating more inferiority around them. This is another type of false measurement, making others around them smaller so that they are adequate in comparison. It is much easier to accept inferiority of self when there is no one around you bettering themselves. After all, there is strength in numbers. Be aware of these people in your life. But more importantly, be aware of these traits in yourself. I am not suggesting removing these people from your life. Should you find that you possess the ability to lose weight through some of the tools in this book, allow others to see your abilities, but be willing to share your ability with them, which brings me to my next point; inspiration.

Inspiration

Do not mistake measuring yourself against others with drawing inspiration from others. There is no wrongdoing in looking at someone else who encapsulates an ability that you are trying to develop. It is said the LeBron James looked up to Michael Jordan growing up. If he were to have succumbed to Jordan's reputation of "The Greatest of All

Time", we may never have witnessed the development of "The King". Is LeBron as good as or better than Jordan? That's a topic that will be discussed for years to come, with supporters on both sides of the panel. What is certain, LeBron was able to study and learn the personality traits of someone who has accomplished what he wanted to accomplish, and implement them with a personal touch.

If you observe someone with the traits that embody the type of person you would like to realize, study them, then implement them through the tools that are provided in this book. Should you find that studying those traits provides you with the ability to realize the true version of yourself, without the self-imposed limitations of your former self-image, share your experiences with others if they are willing to learn them. The ability to live a healthy life in a body that is comfortable to live it in is not a commodity. This ability is unlimited and already exists in each and every one of us. All you have to do is realize it.

Chapter Five

Out with the Old...

It may be of notice to you that often in this text, I repeatedly use the terms "logically", "realistically", "reasonably", and the like. There is a good reason for this. There are only so many entries in the thesaurus when looking for substitutions of the word "rationally".

If the servo-mechanism, or subconscious mind, is an impersonal, goal-striving machine which acts accordingly to the current self-image system you hold, then rational thinking, supplied by the conscious mind can act as the control knob to this machine. With your conscious experience of past events, your self-image has been dictated to you. It is only fair then to assume that conscious thought can change your reaction patterns to given events. For example, how many times in your history of attempting to lose weight have you convinced yourself that is was ok to overeat, or eat something that you feel would have negative consequences regarding your weight? What experience has taught me is that at no time was that one experience going to dismantle your efforts in losing weight. However, we tend to think irrationally when these mishaps occur. We are inclined to think "Well, I blew it today." While it doesn't seem like much, what a statement like this often leads to is

"I'll get started again on Monday." What happens next? A series of indulgences, all of which trigger negative emotions within you regarding how you perceive your ability to lose weight. At this point, it is likely to find yourself in such a negative state of mind, having dug yourself even a larger hole to climb out of, that you rarely do "…get started again on Monday."

Rational Thinking – A Tool for Success

The previous is a very common example that I hear from my clients every day. More so, I have experienced this situation myself. This cycle happens over and over again throughout the course of a dieter's life. It is essential to break this cycle, and the tool to do it is rational thinking. If we were to interrupt this cycle at the point of inception, in this case, just after the dieting mishap occurred, and just before the surrendering white flag of "Well, I blew it today", the subsequent negative events may never have taken place. Suppose you had replaced the phrase "Well, I blew it today", with "I can make up for that mistake throughout the day, or work it off at the gym." By infusing truthful, rational thinking into the situation, you would be able to immediately correct your course, avoiding the subsequent downward spiral of events that lead to you "digging yourself a hole", as displayed in Figure 8. Rational Thinking Tool.

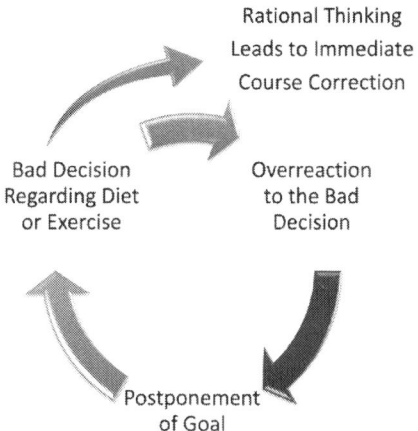

Figure 8. Rational Thinking Tool

At this point, we will introduce the next component of our formula. Rational Thinking by the Conscious Mind, fed to the Imagination will produce a goal or target that is communicated through the Self-Image which is translated as a work order for the Servo-Mechanism, which is illustrated in Figure 9. The Formula.

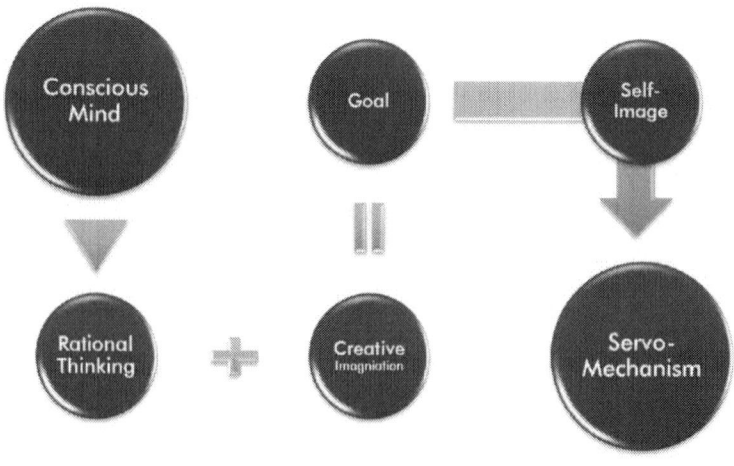

Figure 9. The Formula

Gold Digger

Any skill that is developed and polished is done so by the process of trial and error, or negative feedback, and the subsequent construction of a plan to correct the course so the error does not occur again. For those of you who have swung a golf club at some point in your life more than likely have completely missed the ball on a swing or two. I'd be willing to guess this was a result of lifting your head to see where the ball was going to go before you even made contact, a common ailment in the beginner's golf game. The trial was swinging the golf club. The error was missing the ball due to lifting your head. The irrational decision would be to decide that golf is a stupid game, throw your club to the ground and quit. Infusing the rational thought that you missed the ball because you were not looking at it might give you the patience to try again. Except this time, you correct your course, concentrating on one simple goal; to keep your eyes on the ball. This time, you make contact, taking from the experience the lesson learned. You remember the lesson that you learned; keep your eyes on the ball. You repeat the same series of events over and over again. Before you know it, you are successfully striking the golf ball consistently, and without a single thought paid to watching the ball, because it is habit.

In the process of forming good habits, it is important to realize that just because we learn from past errors doesn't mean we have to carry around all of the excess baggage of that failed event. A way of thinking of this is such as the gold miners of the mid-nineteenth century. When panning for gold, the miner would place a mesh-bottomed pan in the flowing water of a river, pulling it up, and examining it as he shook the excess dirt through the screen. The value lies in the gold, of course, and not the dirt. Learning from past failures should occur in much the same way. When examining our weight loss example, the lesson to be learned was that the concession of "I blew it today" should be replaced with "I can make up for that mistake starting now"; immediate course correction. Given the example of golf, the lesson learned was to "keep your eyes on the ball". These lessons are the gold in the pan. Everything else about these situations, all of the negative emotions experienced at the time of the event, should be tossed back in the proverbially river like the common valueless dirt that they are. There is no reason for you to carry around the left over burden of these past failures when the valuable gold can be extracted and secured alone. In fact, dwelling on past failures is not only time-wasting, but it is threatening to your realization of your true potential. By continually reliving past failures, you just might find yourself evoking those same emotions you experienced when the original failure occurred, causing a false impression on the self-image and dooming you to act in that manner. Always heed the power of your imagination.

Take Your Opponents Head On

Maltz notes two levers for removing obstacles from your path; (1) believing that you are capable of doing your share, exerting a certain amount of independence, and (2) believing that there is something inside of you that should not be allowed to suffer indignities. This couldn't be truer in weight loss.

First of all, you must understand that there is a toll to be paid for losing weight, and that toll is effort. While invariably logical, this concept can often be skewed by hopes for a "magic pill", miraculous surgery, or any other countless "easy buttons" that promise the gift of weight loss with no effort involved. The sooner you accept the fact that these quick fixes don't exist as reality, the sooner your true success can begin. The $60 billion industry, better known as weight loss, has not been built on ethics and truth. Unfortunately, it is predominantly built on fraudulent claims made by charlatans that take advantage of desperate people ready to embrace any possibility of leaving behind those unwanted pounds. Do any of these look familiar?

> *"Lose 30 lbs. in 30 Days!"*
>
> *"Miracle Breakthrough in Weight Loss!"*
>
> *"Eat All You Want and Lose Weight!"*
>
> *"Never Exercise Again!"*

With those simple four statements, we have summarized every faddish weight loss pill, program, cleanse, and equipment marketed to those eager to lose weight on a daily basis. I admit, despite every logical neuron in my brain, I have fallen victim to countless claims that promised me a slim, healthy body with minimal, or no work. Not to belittle those of us who have fallen victim; after all, it is human nature to seek out the pot of gold at the end of the rainbow. Just look at the millions of dollars spent weekly on a one in 76 million chance of winning the Mega Millions Jackpot. However, I will tell you this; I have played the "weight loss miracle lottery" for a long time and never heard of someone winning the jackpot, and certainly never won that jackpot myself. Through my years of education and experience, I have put together several simple, practical behavior modifications that can help reduce the effort that is needed to lose weight, such as eating breakfast, eating small snacks throughout the day, etc. However, I will never tell a client that the pursuit is effortless. I offer my clients personal support, staying in regular contact with them, reminding them of the core elements of this book. But I cannot lose the weight for them. This book outlines how you can reprogram yourself into a habitually healthy person. However, the book will not perform the practical exercises on its own. Therefore, the first question to ask yourself as you prepare to lose weight is "Am I capable of doing my fair share exerting a certain amount of independence?"

The first question is answered, and I assume that you have decided that putting forth an effort is something that you are willing to do. This must be the case, since no magical solutions are hidden in this book. So I pose to you the second question, "Is there an element of you that should not be allowed to suffer one more day with a self-image that affords you overweight or obesity as an acceptable way of life?" I pray that your answer is yes. There is no moral issue to be found with being overweight or normal weight. There is a serious moral issue with believing that you deserve to continually experience the self-imposed limitations that are preventing you from living your life to the fullest. Every day that you resent who you are is a day wasted in your pursuit of becoming the person you are meant to be, in short, happy with yourself.

A Shovel to Uproot Your False Beliefs

Many of the initial components of this book may seem abstract. It is important to construct a strong framework, which can then be used to support the practical tools to help you implement your weight loss success. Let me introduce you to one of those tools. The following is a flow chart, illustrated in Figure 10. Rational Thinking Flowchart, and can be used to identify and eliminate any false beliefs that are holding you back from your weight loss goals.

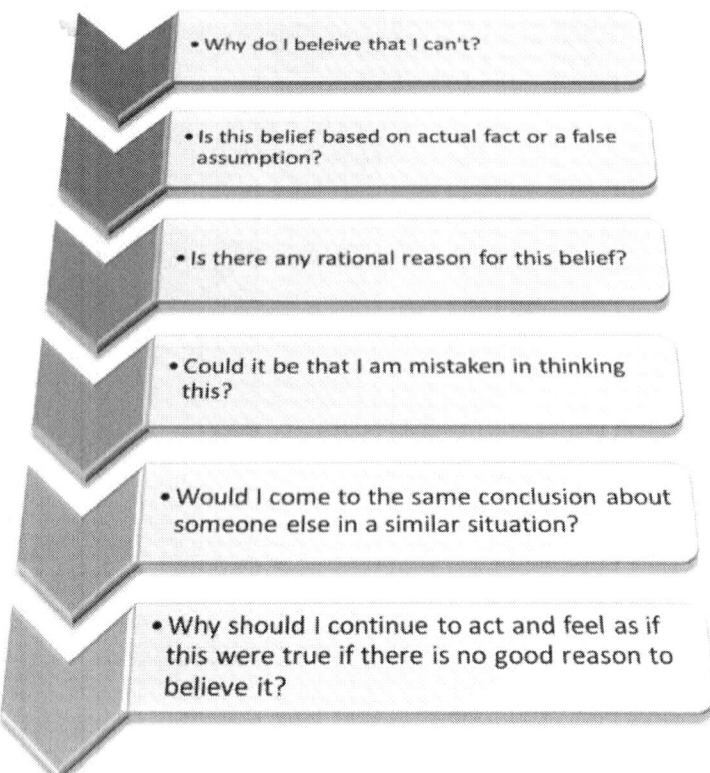

Figure 10. Rational Thinking Flowchart

If at any time while working your way through this flow chart you found yourself coming to the conclusion that you have identified a false belief that has no part being a factor in your self-image, do not get discouraged. Remember, rehashing past failures assures future failures. Instead take the lesson learned, and leave the rest behind. Now let's take that one step further. At this point, replace that feeling of discouragement with anger and indignation. These are powerful emotions that may prove to be very motivating.

These emotions can often be the spark that ignites your unbridled desire to change.

Igniting Your Fire

The pioneers of the science of self-improvement deserve as many gratuitous praises as can be fit into the pages of this book. Classics, such as *Psycho-Cybernetics*, *Think and Grow Rich*, and *The Magic of Believing* were groundbreaking works, and continue to make dramatic impact on the lives of those who embrace their messages. I would like to remind you that this book was never intended to pioneer a new realm of self-improvement. The intention was that this book was to act as a supplement to those classics mentioned above, and the others that I have hastily forgotten to mention. This book's mission is to take those brilliantly devised theses of self-improvement, and apply those principals to weight loss in a practical manner.

This brings us to my next point. As briefly mentioned earlier, Napolean Hill spent a great deal of time discussing the essential inclusion of "desire" in one's pursuit of a goal. Maltz includes *Desire to Change* as the next component of the formula that we have been building throughout the Chapters, as illustrated here in Figure 11. The Formula.

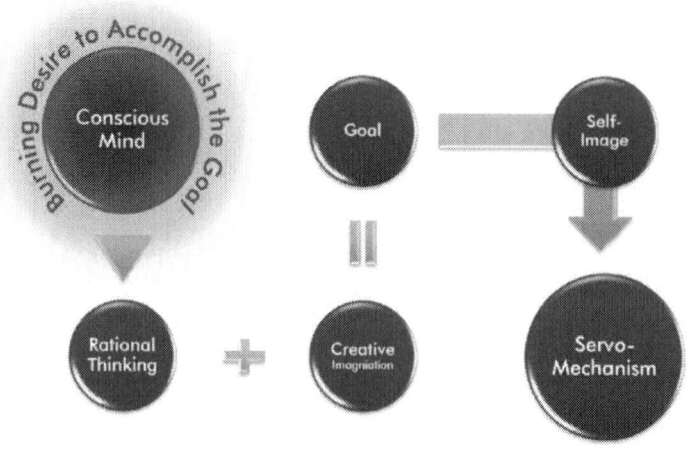

Figure 11. The Formula

Rational Thinking by the Conscious Mind, fueled by Desire to Change, fed to the Imagination will produce a goal or target that is communicated through the Self-Image which is translated as a work order for the Servo-Mechanism.

I remember back to my college days, when a professor of mine repetitively proclaimed a phrase that, at the time, resonated with me; "education leads to behavior modification". This made such sense to me in all its simplicity. If I were to be educated that something that I am doing is inconsistent with my goal, then I will change that behavior. Over time, I have come to realize that this statement lacks at least one major component; *DESIRE*. If you have read the Introduction to this book, you know that I spent my early college career well over 300 lbs. In fact it was at this time that I first heard my professor preach about education and behaviors. Perhaps it was because I was obese and had already defined a clear cut goal in my head to lose weight, and had developed a burning desire to reach that goal, that I overlooked the omission of such a vital factor of change in his statement. If I were to encounter that professor today, I would be inclined to petition him to amend this phrase to "Education leads to behavior modification, should one possess the desire to modify that behavior." In fact, this thesis resembles a popular paradigm shared by many educators; "motivation, education, action."

This theory of desire has been implemented in many ways over the years. The athletic apparel giant Nike has built an entire culture around their trademarked slogan *"Just Do It"*. While a slogan such as this might be inspirational to some, I assume that there is an unsaid understanding behind it that postulates that the *"It"* that one should *"Just Do"* is being supported by a previously decided desire for that *"It"*. Or maybe it is just a catchy slogan used to sell apparel. Regardless, using the formula that is being constructed throughout this book explains that emotions plus logistics equal results. In this case, the emotion is desire. This desire must be cared for like seed in Springtime; one which you will plant in the soil of your conscious mind, tend to while it takes root, until it reaches the point where it is self-sustaining. This is one mental process that we are all very good at. It might not rear its head as desire, but often as *Worry*.

Worry Your Way to Weight Loss

Let's quickly examine the process of how we worry. At some point in our day, a seed, or idea, is planted into our mind. From this idea, we carefully add the "what if". Without as much effort as the blinking of your eyes, this idea of "what if" flourishes into full-blown panic of a disastrous imminent event. Yet, this remains a simple idea that may or may not come to be. Think about the last time that you worried about something. Did you place any effort at all into developing that idea into anxiety over impending doom? How many times have you heard of an athlete achieving remarkable results all through preliminary contests, only to fail on the big stage? The repetition and concentration on negative goals can manifest itself directly into actual failure.

By examining this process, we can utilize its features into developing desire instead of panic. Use the following tutorial to add fuel to your fire.

1. Decide on a goal.
   In maintaining congruency, we will stick to the goal of weight loss. Your seed has now been planted.
2. Add the "What If."
   It is likely that the seed will lay dormant if nothing is provided for it to grow. This is when you will add the "what if." Ponder the idea. "What if I was able to lose weight?"

3. Add Emotion.

As the seed begins to grow, the process can be expedited by adding emotion. This emotion can be found by utilizing your creative imagination, or "the theater of your mind." Remember, the physiologic body cannot decipher between a real event and a vividly imagined event. Experience the weight loss in your mind over and over again until you experience all of the emotions you would expect to feel as if you had already lost the weight.

If you are going to spend your valuable time worrying, why not change the goal from negative to positive? That single element is the only one that needs changed. Instead of the goal being something negative that might happen, substitute something good that might happen, like weight loss. An important fact to remember, it takes a long season of tending to a seedling, or an immature plant. At times, there will be lack of rain, hot days, and cold nights, not to mention critters that will constantly be picking away at it. Luckily, at some point in the future, that seedling will grow to a strong self-sufficient tree that needs no further nurturing. Your goal is no different. Nourish it with constant repetition of "what if", experienced with added positive emotions. Soon enough, your desire will burn so hot, nothing on the face of the earth will be able to extinguish it.

Chapter Six

Go with Your Gut

I have presented you with several techniques regarding how to generally develop a goal. To be honest, goal development is a science, in and of itself. Volumes have been written on proper goal setting, with subsequent elaboration of objectives to reach that goal. I view this topic to carry so much importance in successful weight loss that I have dedicated an entire module of my Zero Resistance Weight Loss System specifically to the development of my clients' goals and objectives. To recount these techniques within the confines of this book is an insurmountable task, however, a brief checklist has been provided to you in the following Chapter. Let it suffice for now to say that you have a goal, which is to lose weight. This Chapter is dedicated to avoiding one of the deadliest sins of weight loss.

You have pondered the idea of losing weight. You have placed careful consideration on whether or not that goal is suitable to you, and whether or not you are willing to pay the toll to reach the destination. You have fertilized your goal with emotion, building immeasurable desire. You have more than likely even put forth a down payment of effort over the years in attempts to reach your goal. So why haven't you done so already. One main reason might be the sin of second-guessing.

Four Phases of Learning

There is no variation of how a human being learns to complete a task, regardless of what that task may be. We will pass through four separate phases while developing any skill set to completion; that is to assume we will reach completion. Very often, we set out to learn a new skill, but get lost along the way, getting stuck in one of these phases.

Phase One: Unconscious Incompetence

This may be difficult to recall, however, there was a point in your life that your body weight did not concern you. Try to recollect this time. This would be prior to you...

...ever going on a diet.

...ever looking at nutrition label with the intent of deciphering a serving size, counting a calorie, a gram of carbohydrates, protein, or fat.

...ever engaging in physical activity with the single purpose of burning off calories or fat.

You get the idea. For some of you, it may be prior to getting married; for others, maybe sometime in childhood. For those lucky ones, it may be a recent discovery that weight loss is something that you may benefit them. Nonetheless, each and every one of us has come from a point in our life's timeline that no such goal of weight loss existed.

I believe it is safe to assume that if no goal of weight loss currently existed, then there would be no point in initiating the development of a skill set that would allow us to reach that goal. This is *Unconscious Incompetence*. At this point, you do not know if you have the ability to lose weight for no other reason than you just haven't tried. You might also think of someone in this stage that has never picked up a guitar. If you were to ask them if they could play guitar, an adequate response would be "I don't know. I've never tried."

Phase Two: Conscious Incompetence

Back to you, if you are reading this book, I assume that you have decided at some point that weight loss is a goal that suits you. This might also be from a time in your past that has been long since forgotten. Unfortunately, this is a phase that many of us will get stuck in.

When attempting to accomplish a goal, such as weight loss, a certain skill set must be developed to progress. For example...

> ...you learn to decipher a Nutrition Facts Panel.

...you begin to memorize the calorie count in certain foods that you eat frequently.

...you mentally calculate about how many calories you burn when exercising.

You are not very good at any of these skills as of yet. In fact, you might be downright terrible. In our example of playing the guitar, this phase would be entered the first time it was picked up and strummed. You've watched people play in the past. Hold a few fingers in the proper configuration, strum with the other hand, and a beautiful melody of sound waves fill the air. It doesn't look that hard. But it is. You awkwardly place your fingers on the frets, forcefully strum with the other hand, and the wailing of painful "notes" penetrates your ears.

Again, in weight loss, many of us get stuck in this stage. We bounce from diet to diet, pill to pill, exercise routine to exercise routine, never mastering a single skill that would actually benefit our attempts in shedding pounds. This phase is extremely frustrating, as our labors produce no reward. I often explain this to my clients using the backdrop of the American financial crisis. We are a society that not only desires, but has come to expect to be able to "buy now, pay later." When we see something we want, we quickly dive into our wallets, remove a piece of plastic, sliding it through a machine, and never think twice about it. If I may, I would like to recommend a shift in this paradigm. Instead of looking for weight loss now, and pay for it later, such as with a magic pill, think of weight loss like a layaway plan. Your small payments of effort over time will eventually lead to your reward, should you be timely and consistent with your payments.

Phase Three: Conscious Competence

The transition from the second to third stage occurs gradually over time, and may not be noticeable in the present. While there is no change in the amount of effort that is being devoted, however, the dividends are beginning to come in. In weight loss, this can be characterized by, after trying countless meal plans, exercise routines, and the like; you have finally found something that works. The result of your efforts is dropping a few pounds. You begin to polish your new found skill, making it your own, fine-tuning every aspect of it until it is a well-oiled machine. In considering our guitar example, the practice, or effort remains the same. Except now, when you consciously place your fingers on the frets, it begins to feel natural. Using your other hand, you strum gracefully, extracting melodious sounds from the piece of formed, hollowed out wood.

If you are lucky enough to reach this phase, you may find that fate is much like that of the second; a failure to progress to the next. While you have developed a skill or two that will help you towards your goal, by no means have you constructed the full skill set which will allow you the path of *Zero Resistance*. This may foster from…

...fatigue from putting forth effort, demonstrated as,

> *"I just can't make it to the gym anymore."*
>
> *"I'm starving. I can't survive on lettuce and chicken."*

...resentment from results not coming quick enough, demonstrated as,

> *"I can't believe that I worked out every day this week and only lost a half of a pound."*

...complacency with how far you've come, demonstrated as,

> *"I set out to lose fifty pounds, but I am pretty happy with the thirty I've already lost."*

...loss of desire for where you planned on going, demonstrated as,

> *"This diet isn't worth me skipping any more dinners out with my friends."*

It is a shame for someone to get stuck in this phase. This is where you would find most of your yo-yo dieters. They are so close to progressing to the next phase and don't even realize it. I do not intend to voice my opinions in this book on what type of diet should be followed, and which should be avoided. If you have found any type of diet to be successful in the past, and as long as it is not an endangerment to any component of your health, then I would support you being on that diet for the time being. The focus of this book is to help you progress from this third phase of success with effort, to the next phase of success without effort. However, I will infuse this caveat. In learning to play the guitar, the general means to the end is practice. But professionals will tell you that certain methods provide much faster results than others. Losing weight is no different. Several methods of dietary restriction, physical activity inclusion, etc., are much more effective, efficient, and safer than other alternatives. Be cautious which method you choose to lose weight, and do so with the support of a professional.

At this point I would like to personally offer to help you out, and remind you that I am only an email, phone call, or website comment away. I have become fluent in building cohesive and successful weight loss programs for hundreds of people. The wonder of technology has removed the barrier of location from preventing you in contacting me. The intermingling of nutritional science, exercise science, and cognitive science ultimately leads to an unparalleled probability of successful weight loss. This information is yours for the taking. You simply need to ask.

Phase Four: Unconscious Competence

This phase promises the reward of experiencing the emotions felt only after the greatest of accomplishments. Picture Eric Clapton, or the late Jimi Hendrix on stage. Do you think a single conscious thought ever crossed their mind when a guitar was in their hands? Do you think any effort is placed on "holding down these fingers", or "strumming with this intensity?" Of course not. The competence of their skill set is derived from their servo-mechanism. The complex series of movements that produce that sound originate directly from habit. They were not born with this talent. It was cultivated, just like any other skill set must be.

This holds true for the skill set required for losing weight, and living a healthy life. It is with the practice of the applications in this book that you can master losing weight, making a habit out of healthy living, totally avoiding the use of will power, dropping pound after pound until your goal is reached. However, this model follows the layaway paradigm, not purchasing on credit. You must be willing to form a goal, develop a desire to accomplish it, place effort in learning the skills in this book, and practice them. Take action. Learning a new task, such as weight loss, is no different from playing the guitar, driving a car, or learning to tie your shoes. Every skill can be developed to a point of unconscious competence, or *Zero Resistance*.

Make it Right

As posed in *Psycho-Cybernetics*, "… the truth is that there are very few inherently right or wrong decisions. Instead, we make decisions, then make them right." This rings true with weight loss. How much time have you spent preparing to take action? How much time have you spent giving yourself the excusal from effort for an entire week by saying "I'll start on Monday"? If you are to embrace what this book provides, you should never have to waste another day planning to take action. You simply WILL take action, with the confidence that if you make a mistake, you can simply correct it and move on. All of this can be accomplished in that creative part of the brain. There are three principals to adhere to at all costs, and in doing so, can free your goals to take flight, instead of lying dormant while you ponder how to take action.

Never Second Guess Your Goal

We discussed this earlier, so I will keep this segment brief. You have a goal. You want to lose weight. You have spent time deciding that you have the ability to complete it, and likewise have the desire to accomplish it. You have an idea of what you need to do to get started. You've even taken the first step, whether in a right or wrong direction doesn't matter at this point.

From this point on, a single moment should not be spent, nor the slightest amount of energy wasted, questioning the value, purpose, or validity of that goal. It was important to you. It is important to you. Never let negative emotions trigger the downward spiral that leaves your goal gathering dust. Effort must be made to achieve a level of unconscious competence and *Zero Resistance*. Do not carry around the burden of negative "what ifs" while you are walking your journey.

Live in the Now

How many different ways are there to say "live in the now?" Countless philosophers gained worldly notoriety professing…

> "…*The past is a guidepost, not a hitching post.*" – L. Thomas Holdcroft

> "…*Forever is composed of nows.*" – Emily Dickinson

Yet, it is the thought and work of Ralph Waldo Emerson that I find to be most enlightening:

> "…*With the past, I have nothing to do; nor with the future. I live now.*"

> "…*Finish each day and be done with it. You have done what you could; some blunders and absurdities have crept in; forget them as soon as you can. Tomorrow is a new day; you shall begin*

*it serenely and with too high a spirit to be
encumbered with your old nonsense."*

Your past serves one purpose, to provide insight into what
you could have changed to do better. You cannot change
these events. You've overeaten at lunch. Why? Because you
did not eat breakfast. You just ate a pound of spaghetti.
Why? Because you have been eating no carbohydrates for
the past week and found that it was much too difficult to
maintain that type of diet long-term. Take the lesson
learned, and leave the past in the past.

Why waste time pondering what the future holds? Will you
lose ten pounds by next month if you follow your diet plan
and maintain your activity level? It is unknown. But one
thing is for sure. You will NOT lose ten pounds this month
by not monitoring your diet and maintaining your physical
activity level. While we cannot predict the future, we can
shape the events about to unfold by the actions we take now,
based on the lessons we have learned in the past. The funny
thing about the future is that it will never be reached. Just as
you think you are one moment closer, that moment changes
to the present. There is no escaping it, so make the best of it.

Make Every Crisis Take a Number

With this fast-paced world, there is an unadulterated
emphasis being placed on the ability to multitask. Whether
or not we have perfected this skill is arbitrary, as we are
expected to be able to do it. The essence of multitasking is

found in the pages of this book. You are training your servo-mechanism to be able to handle situations out of habit. You are training your servo-mechanism to make decisions and take actions throughout your day to assure a healthy lifestyle. Of course, as you know, there will come times that an obstacle drops in front of you, and your servo-mechanism will be unprepared to handle this event. The only reasons that this can occur is that you have not experienced that situation before, or have not learned from the experience that has provided the lesson in the past. It is imperative during the occurrences of these events that we place the obstacles in a single file line, making them each take a number.

Each obstacle, or crisis situation, which we will discuss further in a later Chapter, possesses its own level of importance. To be more precise, each crisis situation will cause more or less damage than the next if handled out of order. While on your path towards your weight loss goal, issues are destined to arise, where your servo-mechanism does not yet have the necessary information to handle it on its own. You must now institute your conscious mind and creative mechanism to determine how to best handle that situation. Don't worry. This will be a valuable learning experience for the next time it arises. When several of these issues arise at one time, the mood can become quite frustrating. It is not that you cannot handle the workload. The frustration arises because you have not assigned these obstacles an order by which you will handle them.

Work your way through the following dilemma. You sit at work in the early afternoon looking forward to leaving at three o'clock when the following thoughts strike you. You have no food in your house to prepare for dinner. Your oldest son has to be at baseball practice at 4:30. Your daughter has to be at gymnastics by five. Now, your youngest son calls to tell you about a school project that is due tomorrow that is worth half of his grade. All of this on top of the fact that you truly had every intention and desire to make it to the gym to log a few miles on the treadmill. Anxiety starts to build. Soon you find yourself paralyzed by the army of crises surrounding you. No one of these situations is enough to make you wince on its own. And if each of these situations were to have presented themselves in a timely fashion, there is no doubt that you could have accomplished them. But they didn't present themselves timely, so you must make them timely. Sort through them in order of importance, or in order of how much consequence the incompletion of the task would bear. Your family has to eat, so you plan to get to the store directly after work to pick up just the essentials. You will then get home, unpack the groceries, while leaving out a box of whole wheat spaghetti, a couple of chicken breasts and a bag of frozen broccoli. You've made better meals, but it will do. Back into the car with your son and daughter for a swift delivery to their respective practices. Back home to prepare dinner, an easy task, allowing you to help your son with his project simultaneously; an example of your servo-mechanism at work. Dinner is ready, and can be reheated when you get home. Back into the car to pick up your children from practice. Home again and dinner is served. After another hour of finishing up the school work, your tasks are complete, all except the treadmill. It's getting late, and a drive to the gym is out of the question. You decide, using your creative mechanism, that walking a few laps around the block will suffice.

Admittedly, it is easy for me to pose a fictitious situation that I was in control of the entire time. But you have been in a similar situation. How much time we waste building the frustration instead of taking on the tasks one step at a time. Even if you hadn't fit your walk in, is that the end of the world? No. It was simply a reason to learn the lesson at hand. Maybe tomorrow you'll walk in the morning.

Chapter Seven

Don't Worry, Be Happy

During my initial consultation with a new client, I will ask them an extremely loaded question; "What do you want to get out of my services?" The answers vary greatly, but each one has a common thread. Their answers are a clue into how much thought they have put in to developing their goal. If I receive an answer such as "I want to lose twenty-five pounds over the next three months", or "I want to be able to get off of my cholesterol medication within the year", I know that I am dealing with someone that has an advanced system of goal development. However, I often hear answers that more resemble "I just want to be skinny." This is a parallel of what Maltz records as "I just want to be happy", and goes on to explain how an overly generalized goal is an often used excuse for a poorly devised goal.

Every goal we set for our body weight, or for that matter any issue dealing with personal health improvement, is a reflection of what we hold to be a physical representation of our happiness. In essence, our weight loss goal will provide us with happiness, and every care should be taken to process each goal so it will deliver us happiness accordingly. However, the end result of happiness is a side effect of achieving any such more specific goal, and to state a goal as general as so is to serve a great disservice to you chances of success.

Setting Goals for Guaranteed Success

A simple tool that can be used to evaluate your goals lies within the word *SMART*. I cannot take credit for the development of this tool, and further cannot tell you who should be given the credit. What I can tell you is that this tool is frequently prescribed to those who have trouble being concise while goal setting. This is a very small part of my Zero Resistance Goals and Objective Building Module that I have extracted to help you start building your foolproof path to success.

S – Specific

> Make sure that every goal you set has a high level of specificity to it. For example, *losing weight*, instead of *being healthy or happy*.

M – Measurable

> Take it a step further now. Assign a measurable component to your goal. For example, *losing twenty-five pounds*, instead of *losing weight*.

A – Attainable

> Evaluate your goal to assure that it is realistic. While I admire those who "shoot for the

stars", setting goals outside of the realm of physical possibility are never productive. Twenty-five pounds of weight loss is an attainable goal, assuming that you are willing to provide ample time, which we will get to in a moment.

R – Relevant

As I mentioned earlier in the Chapter, the main purpose of any goal we set is that it will provide us with a level of happiness. If being overweight plagues you with a level of unhappiness, losing twenty-five pounds should very well provide you with happiness, and is therefore relevant to your cause.

T – Time Sensitive

Lastly, it is imperative that your goal be time-sensitive. A goal with an open-ended time frame welcomes procrastination. We can solidify this weight loss goal into "I want to lose twenty-five pounds in three month".

All of the elements of a strong goal are now present. It is now imperative to take action, as the procurement of happiness lies within accomplishing our goals.

The Art and Science of Happiness

It is important to understand that happiness carries with it no moral value. Happiness is not a commodity, to be hoarded by a chosen minority. It can be manifested in all walks of life, achieved by the most common of common people. All that is needed is a clear cut goal, where accomplishment of that goal will undoubtedly provide you with a physical asset or personal attribute that you place a certain value on. At the same time, if a state of happiness can be achieved prior to goal achievement, that emotional status alone may be enough to reduce the effort needed to achieve those goals.

The Chicken or the Egg?

It is well documented in medical research that experience of the state of happiness has a profound impact on physical health, both chronic and acute. In the September 1986 issue of *Psychosomatic Medicine*, researchers concluded that blood pressure is significantly lower when a feeling of happiness is induced, when compared to emotional states of anxiety and anger. In fact, numerous studies have proposed and supported that all of the internal organs can optimally function when a state of happiness is being experienced. Additionally, happiness has been shown to heighten sensations of vision, hearing, taste, and touch. As a side note, it also has been supported in literature that heightened taste sensation can lead to expedited satiation, or fullness, during meals. This in itself may provide a subconscious relief to overeating.

In the American Psychological Association's *Psychological Bulletin* published in November 2005, researchers examined data from several research articles. These data suggest that "happiness is associated with and precedes numerous successful outcomes, as well as behaviors paralleling success." Furthermore, "...many of the desirable characteristics, resources, and successes correlated with happiness." These two statements are encouraging findings, explaining that while success breeds happiness, a lesser known factor is clear; happiness breeds success as well. I feel inclined to share the words of Sir Arthur Helps, "Rien ne réussit comme le success", meaning *"Nothing succeeds like success."*

What a remarkable cycle of events, as illustrated in Figure 12. Happiness-Success Cycle, that can take place. It is logical to assume that achieving your goals will bring you happiness. But have you ever thought that happiness would help you to achieve those goals. The wonderful part of this cycle is the simplicity of it. You can enter the cycle by achieving a goal that will provide you with a level of happiness. Additionally, you can manifest happiness through the use of your creative imagination to help you achieve your goals. Once in the cycle, the sequence of events will carry you from success to happiness, and back to more success, over and over again. If happiness is a chicken and success is an egg, we would be foolish to pay a care to which comes first.

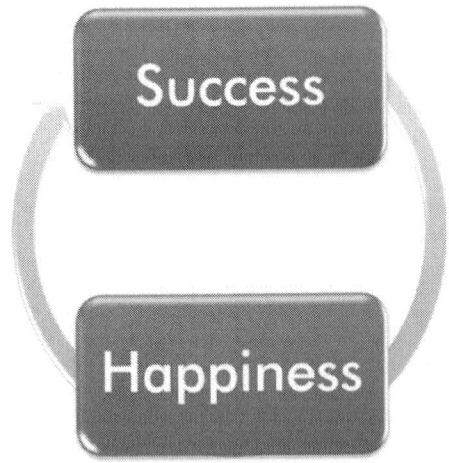

Figure 12. Happiness-Success Cycle

Don't Cry Over Spilled Milk

We don't jump in our cars for our morning drive to work and say "I hope I don't wreck my car." We simply focus on the goal, "I will drive to work." Weight loss should be approached the same way. The following sections will illustrate guaranteed ways to experience unhappiness. Learn from the mistakes and capture their lessons.

Happy Being Unhappy

We all know someone who relishes in their own misery. Call them what you will, but a common sarcastic moniker is "martyr". These people seek out unhappiness, therefore providing themselves a perverse sense of satisfaction; always putting others first. That act may sound saintly; however, they are quick to let you know what they just did for you.

Take, for example, a time that your daughter hit the winning home run in her softball game. When asked what she wants to do to celebrate, she says she wants to order a pizza for dinner. You are in the middle of your best weight loss attempt yet, and you are sure that the mental impact of one slice will lead to you eating many, many more. There are plenty of options for you to take. You could plan to eat something completely different. You could apply rational thinking and good sense, filling up on a salad, affording you the ability to limit your pizza to one or two slices. However, you decide to take "the high road", offering to just eat the pizza because your family wants it, and seeing them happy is most important, and you are willing to sacrifice for it. You are now in a negative state of mind, which will commonly lead to negative consequences. You overeat. Your frustration builds. You begin to question your ability to achieve your goal, since occasions like this always seem to arise when you are trying to lose weight.

This is just one type of example where attempting to provide someone else with happiness had a negative consequence. You feel perversely vindicated that you were "forced" to absorb the negative consequence of eating the pizza. You used the idea of providing your daughter with happiness as a chance to provide yourself with feeling like a martyr, which ultimately led to everyone's unhappiness. This is a dangerous cycle to find yourself in; where unhappiness becomes the goal.

Looking Forward to Being Happy

Dale Carnegie said "One of the most tragic things I know about human nature is that all of us tend to put off living. We are all dreaming of some magical rose garden over the horizon - instead of enjoying the roses that are blooming outside our windows today." The future holds your goal's accomplishment. Your future holds the "new and improved you" that you want to be; the you of today, only slightly slimmer. It is obvious that achieving that goal will bring you happiness. But that goal that lies in the future will never be realized if you do not spend every present moment accomplishing the practical objectives that will get you there. These objectives might be monitoring your portion size, logging thirty minutes of exercise every day, concentrating on replacing refined starches with whole grains, etc. Each one of these objectives, no matter how trivial they seem, should provide you with an equity share of the happiness that lies in the future. Experience the emotion that comes with each and every one of these accomplishments. Do not fall victim to minimizing their importance by saying things like...

> *"...I lost a few pounds, but I have a long way to go."*

> *"...I got my thirty minutes in on the treadmill today, but I have another ninety to get in this week."*

These are prime examples of minimizing the importance of your journey towards your goal. It is simply impossible for you to lose all the weight that you want to today. It is simply impossible to fit all the exercise you need to accomplish your goal today. Instead, relish what you can and have accomplished.

I will leave this section with a simple analogy. Your weight loss journey is a marathon. Each stride you take in this marathon is of equal importance. It is human nature to view those last ten strides as monumental. We have been taught that the happiness of crossing that finish line is immeasurable. But I ask you this. Were those first ten strides any less important? Without those first ten strides, the last ten still leaves you short of your goal. Enjoy each and every stride as an accomplishment of its own equal importance.

It's Nothing Personal

We all experience petty annoyances throughout the day. Our reaction to these petty annoyances is dictated by two things; (1) the emotional state we find ourselves in, and (2) how we perceive the intent of the annoyance. Often times, the prior will directly affect the latter. Here is an example. You normally get off of work at three o'clock, which is normally followed by a quick trip to the gym to fit in your workout and relieve some stress. Unfortunately, your boss asked you to stay until five (annoyance number one), because you are the only person he feels is capable of completing this project on time. After all, that's why he made you the office manager. Upon entering the gym, you remember why you always go at three. It is packed, and not a treadmill to be found (annoyance number two). As your frustration builds, you belligerently stomp to the one elliptical machine that is available, sandwiched in between two people who have obviously been there a while, as the sweat is dripping off of them (annoyance number three). Only five minutes in to your workout, the sweaty man next to you happens to inadvertently brush against you (annoyance number four). You abruptly jump off the elliptical machine, grab your keys, and walk right out the door.

So there you are; extremely frustrated and driving home with angst, honking at anyone who dares drive within three car lengths. Worst of all, you didn't accomplish your objective; to exercise and relieve stress. And why? Admittedly, these annoyances can get to the best of us on any given day, but the sequence of events may have been interrupted, or at least the emotional attachment and sabotage that came with it, with some simple rationale thinking. You were already frustrated having to stay at work late. However, it is reasons like that that got you the promotion in the first place. The gym was packed when you arrived, and you were stuck using a piece of equipment you are not familiar with, the elliptical machine. But everyone didn't gather there waiting for you to pull into the parking lot and rush to beat you to the treadmills. It's five o'clock and most people are just getting out of work. The man next to you brushes against you. There is a very slim chance that he actually wanted to use your arm as a sweat towel. Isn't he there simply trying to do the same thing you are?

Fact Versus Opinion

As described in the previous example, you can see that impressing your opinion onto, or your impression of, a situation can be hazardous. Epictetus said "Men are disturbed not by the things that happen, but by their opinion of the things that happen." Take this story, for example. You have been successfully losing weight for the months. It's time to go the mall and pick up a few new outfits that will better compliment the slimmer you. You choose a few outfits and head to the fitting room. Starting with one size down from your regular clothing, you realize it is still too large; what a great feeling it is! After trying the next size down, you feel the outfit might be just a little too snug, but you really like it and know that it will soon fit you just fine. You exit the fitting room to get a better look at it in the full size mirror. While examining yourself in the outfit, you notice two sales clerks looking at you but talking too softly for you to decipher what they are saying. Almost in tears, you speed off into the changing room, put on your old baggy clothes and head home.

What is your perception of what just happened? Do you assume that the two clerks were making fun of you for having tried on an outfit that may have been too tight? That is one opinion. I repeat…OPINION. What if I were to tell you the clerks were discussing the other colors of the outfit that you were wearing, since they thought it looked so good on you they wanted to suggest some alternatives? Now you are left with the same old clothing, teary eyes, and a severely dented self-image, all because you impressed your opinion on the situation.

"X'ing Out" of Unhappiness

Computers have gone from luxury to necessity in recent history, as with exposure to the internet, and the knowledge it has to offer, has become a daily event. With that in mind, we have all been exposed to "pop-ups"; those uninvited, annoying little advertisements that, well, pop up on our screens while browsing your favorite websites. In fact, we have become so accustom to them, it is rare that the message ever has a chance to be read, as we quickly move the mouse arrow to the right hand corner and click on the "X'. No effort is used in removing these pop-ups. It has become a habit to "X-out" the negative.

You can use this same method to learn a new habit of removing the everyday occurrences that stand in the way of your happiness. Of course, all habits are built with a little effort and repetition. With that repetition, the effort diminishes rapidly, as our servo-mechanism begins to take over, just as it has as you close those nasty pop-ups. Let's use the above sections and examples as a display.

In the section titled *Happy Being Unhappy*, I introduced you to a situation where a celebratory event was plagued by your self-righteousness and martyrdom. If at any time during this series of events you would have been able to say...

> "...*This is my daughter's moment. It has nothing to do with my diet.*"

> "...*The goal of me losing weight will bring me happiness, but celebrating my daughter's victory can do the same.*"

...then you would have "X'd" out of the negative.

In the section titled *Looking Forward To Being Happy*, I presented to you the idea of minimizing your small successes, in the shadow of the great success you are looking forward to. Instead of saying...

> "...*I lost a few pounds, but I have a long way to go.*"

say...

> "*A few more pounds lost. I'm on my way to my goal, a little closer every day!*"

Instead of saying...

> "...*I got my thirty minutes in on the treadmill today, but I have another ninety to get in this week.*"

say...

"Another thirty minutes down, and two miles closer to my goal!"

In the section titled *It's Nothing Personal*, the annoying series of events leading up to your abrupt exit of the gym thwarted every goal you entered with. None of those events constituted a personal vendetta against you. There was no personal intention involved. Yet, it is common for us to experience sequences of events like this and assume the world is against us. Honestly, there's a high probability not a single person in the gym even noticed you until you made a spectacle of yourself leaving. Self-pity can escalate a minor annoyance into a complete meltdown.

Finally, in *Fact Versus Opinion*, you were confronted with the idea that your personal opinion of a matter can be very deconstructive, as seen with assuming that the clerks were whispering negative comments about you. If you would have simply "X'd out" your personal opinion, you could have avoided a drastic misunderstanding, a bruised self-image, and had a new outfit all at the same time.

You will be confronted numerous times throughout every day with obstacles ranging greatly in their actual detriment to your goal's accomplishment. By creating a system that allows you to identify when you are experiencing a self-imposed negative emotion, as illustrated in this Chapter, you can then apply a little rational thinking to get right back on track.

Chapter Eight

We are the Champions

Success and failure describe personalities, accommodated by the self-image, built from a foundation of thoughts, bricks of action, and mortar of habits.

Seven Characteristics of Success

Maltz identified seven distinct characteristics of success-type personalities, which conveniently fit into the acronym *SUCCESS,* and illustration of which can be found in Figure 13. Success Acronym.

"S" is for "Sense of Direction"

As a pillar of this book, sense of direction refers to your goal. We have reviewed repetitively that the servo-mechanism was built to perform one action, goal-striving. It is completely objective, impersonal, and nonjudgmental. It will complete any task assigned to it, as long as the goal is consistent with the self-image.

Imagine driving cross-country, from the east coast to the west. Even without a map or navigation system, probability is high that you could accomplish this. There are highways signs that can keep you on track. Now imagine doing so as if all signs had been removed. This might take your chances from probable to improbable very quickly.

Imagine that the east coast is the present. The west coast, your weight loss goal. The highway markers are the series of successful objective accomplishments made along the way. It is easy to become lost if your journey consists of only the goal. At times, this goal can be too far to see. But there are numerous markers that we can keep our eyes on, being confident that we are on the right track. The person who reminds themselves "I have to lose fifty pounds" will have far less success that the person who reminds themselves "I have to pack my healthy lunch today", "I need to get my servings of fruit in today", or "I need to fit in one more hour of exercise this week.".

"U" is for "Understanding"

In order to overcome any obstacle in the way of your weight loss, you must first have a general understanding of that obstacle. It is said that the origin of fear is the unknown. Why are children afraid of the dark? Because they do not know what it contains. Why do we fear the holidays when we are attempting to lose weight? Because our control over the events in front of us dissipates dramatically. This fear is futile. The holidays will come regardless of it. Accepting failure and leaving your goal lying dormant during the holidays is silly, since just as you are not sure if the holidays will be filled with cookie trays and indulgence, you can be sure that the majority of the holiday season can be spent following that same healthy routine that you have been all along.

It is also imperative that we have an understanding of where our successes and failures are originating from. In the following example, we have one executive who holds regular meeting with his employees. During these meetings, he encourages open discussions about what is working, and what is not, without the employees feeling threatened if having to present bad news. On the other hand, we have an executive who runs things from the top, implementing schemes as he sees fit. No employee dare tell him that something isn't working, as they were all his ideas to begin with. Which better embodies the success-type personality? Without the knowledge that can be provided from his employees' feedback, the second executive lacks the negative feedback necessary to correct the course.

It is no different when attempting to lose weight. Do not blame the scale for your weight gain despite all of your exercise. You may find it more beneficial to develop an understanding that your diet has been holding you back. Likewise, do not credit the "magic pill" you are taking with your success at losing weight. It would have not been possible without the efforts of your diet and physical activity. In another common theme, you very well know that the holiday season does not have a magic power that forces you to eat too much every day, at every hour of the day. Maybe your family is not excessively supportive of your goal. Does that mean they are force-feeding you fast food and potato chips? Give credit where credit is due, and blame where it is warranted, whether in success or failure. But be warned, as soon as you are to give the credit or blame to external sources outside of your control, you lose the ability to create our own future in goals being achieved. If you believe the weight staring back at you on your scale is the sole criteria to whether or not you are succeeding, you have given away your control. If you believe that the weight loss pill you are taking is the only reason you are losing weight, you have given away your control. If you believe that there is not point to watching your diet over a six-week holiday season, from mid-November to late-December, you have given away control.

I have reviewed a few common examples of understanding the obstacles of losing weight; over awareness of the scale, use of weight loss supplements, giving up over the holidays, unsupportive families. Take a moment to ponder your own obstacles of losing weight. Do you have an understanding of the truth behind them?

"C" is for "Courage"

Now that you have acknowledged the facts about why you are or are not achieving your goals, you must find the courage to act, or continue to act on that knowledge. This courage usually happens in two phases.

In the first phase, you must find the courage to accept responsibility for the facts at hand. It is only at this time that you will have true understanding of the obstacles. Do you have the courage to accept the responsibility that only you are in control of your day to day decisions? Your scale does not mock you. It simply reports to you the force of gravity that is enacted on the mass of your body. Note that I said mass, not fat. The body is made up of numerous components, with fat being only one of them. There is also bone, muscle, water, organs, etc. Is it possible that your exercise and healthy eating is actually working, even though the scale hasn't budged? Maybe you have increased your muscle mass. Maybe you are retaining water from yesterday's salty dinner. Likewise, do you have the courage to accept responsibility that just because you have holiday cookies in the house, that you don't have to eat them every day? How about the courage to acknowledge that your family is not out to sabotage you, but do not want to risk offending you by encouraging you to eat less or exercise more? On a more positive note, do you have the courage to accept responsibility for the good you are doing? Maybe it is your exercise and diet that have yielded a reduction in weight, and not that magic pill. At this point, it is necessary to take your understanding one step further, as no amount of understanding will ever be enough without the courage to accept it.

In the second phase, you must find the courage to take action. These lessons are easy to put into words on these pages, however, practicing them is a much more difficult task. Following phase one, you have found the courage to accept the responsibility for your own actions, and how those actions will impact your health. You must now find the courage to utilize that knowledge to change your behaviors. It is not uncommon to get stuck at this point. It is in our human nature to desire order, organization, and perfection; the desire for everything to fall into place just as we see it happening. The truth is, you must have the courage to fail. Once you acknowledge the fact that perfection is unattainable, a series of temporary failures becomes acceptable. The key to this is having the courage to correct these failures as they occur, one holiday cookie at a time, so to say.

"C" is for "Charity"

Expanding your self-image to a point where it will no longer restrict you from accomplishing your goals is a main facet of this book. The act of charity is a tool that can expand your self-image by leaps and bounds. This act of charity must not be derived from self-deprecation, or feeling that others are superior to you and therefore must be treated as such. And vice versa, this act of charity must not be derived from superiority, or attempting to gain recognition from the act. This act of charity must come from your recognition that each and every one of us is a unique person, each with equal worth, and deserve to be treated as such. In fact, every major religion has this common thread in their golden rule. In Christianity…

> "Teacher, which is the great commandment in the Law?"

> "Jesus said to him, You shall love the LORD your God with all your heart, and with all your mind and with all your soul... and You shall love your neighbor as yourself." - Matthew 22:36-40

In Buddhism...

> "Hurt not others with that which pains yourself or in ways that you yourself would find hurtful. One should seek for others the happiness one desires for one's self" - Udana-Varqa, 5:18

In Islam...

> "Not one of you is a believer until he desires for another that which he desires for himself." - Muhammad, 40 Hadith of an-Nawawi 13

In Judaism,

> "What is hateful to you, DO NOT to your fellow man. That is the law: all the rest is commentary." - Talmud, Shabbat 31a

This list could go on for pages, from Eastern to Western cultures, or in non-religious sects such as Greek philosophy. The meaning of the word Charity has become skewed over generations. True charity is following any golden rule you see fit, as long as it includes recognizing the worth of every person. Should you follow this rule as it was intended, you will undoubtedly come to one conclusion without the least bit of effort; you are worthy to be treated charitably by others, but most importantly, by yourself.

Charity is often viewed as a moral issue. "It is moral to act charitably." I tend to believe that charity is less built in morality and more built in essentiality. It is essential to recognize others, making it essential that we recognize ourselves, and our own purpose. Weight loss is very similar, in this regard. Weight loss in not a moral issue. However, if you fail to recognize your own self-worth, or the worth of reaching your goals, you may find it immoral for you to accomplish your weight loss goal.

"E" is for "Esteem"

Esteem is a factor of success, closely related to charity. In fact, it is its reflection in the mirror. If you are to treat people with respect, simply because they are who they are, you will find that you must treat yourself the same way. If you recall from the previous section, charity should not be acted upon in a manner that causes self-deprecation. This would result in self-disesteem. Regardless of what faith you follow, or do not follow, just as you will never find it written that you should serve only yourself, you will never find it written that you must serve only others.

Many of us, at one time or another, have acted out through martyrdom. In some perverse way, we find some joy in being the person who does for others at the cost of our own happiness. This perverse joy can quickly begin a cycle of self-deprecation, where we find reward in being unhappy. The cost of this reward is self-doubt, leaving us contemplating if we deserve to achieve what we once thought was so important. As Maltz said, "Self-doubt is insidious, and gnaws away at the self-image as cancer eats away at the organs." Should you find that you doubt your own ability to lose weight, you will quickly find that your abilities will crumble.

"S" is for "Self-Confidence"

Developing faith in your ability to achieve your goal, in this case, weight loss, may seem like an insurmountable task. How are you to develop self-confidence when you have been met with nothing but failures? The answer is actually quite simple. Ask yourself one question, "Is it possible for me to lose weight?" When you answer this question, do not include any prejudice of your past experiences. Simply answer as a matter of fact, and science. "Am I able to achieve weight loss?" Of course you are! When your caloric intake is less than your caloric expenditure your body utilizes fat stores to fuel your body. Have you noticed that this is about the third time that I have used this statement in this book? An example of an authoritative figure using repetition to make you believe. You are not an anomaly of science with whom this formula will not work. So why do you lack the confidence to accomplish the task? The answer to this question can also be found quite easily. Your confidence, or lack thereof, is built on upon a series of past successes and failures.

In previous Chapters, I have stressed the importance of learning lessons from the past and leaving the rest behind, taking the gold and leaving the dirt, so to say. If you have found this difficult to do, I encourage you to keep practicing it; however, here is another tool that you can use in the meantime. Your experiencing of a series of small failures has naturally led to a lack of self-confidence. A doughnut for breakfast led to you eating unhealthily the rest of the day, week, or month. A skipped workout led to you not stepping foot on the treadmill until the following Monday. Consequently, this cycle will work in reverse. Every time you experience a success, you add to your self-confidence. With each success, you expand the circumference of your self-image. Pay special attention to each and every success that you have. Visualize your self-image growing, allowing you to set goals that are larger and larger. Every time you eat a piece of fruit instead of a candy bar; every time you make it to the gym; every time you pack you lunch; relish in your success.

"S" is for "Self-Acceptance"

As we conclude the SUCCESS acronym, the final S might as well stand for *SUMMARY* instead of *SELF-ACCEPTANCE*. Self-acceptance combines every other success-type trait into one.

Sense of Direction. Your weight loss goal was chosen a long time ago. You might choose to forget it from time to time, but it will continue to resurface until it is achieved, because you have *accepted* it.

Understanding. Through past success and failure, you are working on developing a thesis as to what can help you lose weight, as well as what hinders you. You are *accepting* the facts of your abilities to lose weight.

Courage. You realize that the knowledge of what needs to be changed is simply not enough. You must act on this knowledge. You *accept* the challenge.

Charity and Esteem. You are treating others charitably, showing them respect, for no other reason than they exist. By treating others charitably, you *accept* that you deserve the same, from others and yourself.

Self-Confidence. You have *accepted* that each of your successes is just as valuable to contributing to your confidence, just as each failure has effortlessly chipped away at it.

Self-Acceptance is just that; the realization that you are who you are. This book will not provide you with super powers that will magically make weight loss suddenly achievable.

The goal is to realize that you have always had the ability to accomplish your weight loss goal; you just haven't realized those abilities yet. To achieve strength, you must first accept that you have been weak. To achieve knowledge, you must first accept that you have been ignorant and naive. To achieve courage, you must first accept that you have been acting in fear.

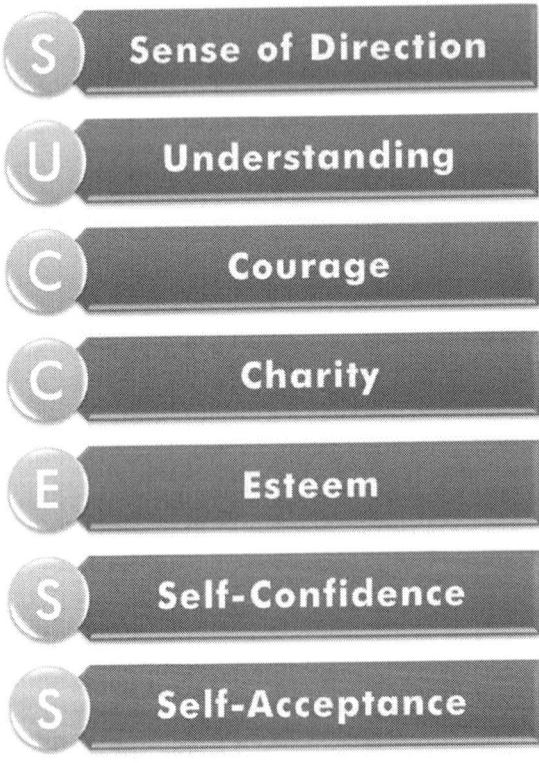

Figure 13. Success Acronym

Chapter Nine

No Time for Losers

Just as successful people can be categorized as having the common traits described in the previous Chapter, there is a similar model for failure-type personalities, which is illustrated in Figure 14. Failure Acronym. And just as engaging in acting out the success characteristics, the ability to recognize the characteristics of failure can stop you from that downward spiral we all know so well.

Seven Characteristics of Failure

"F" is for "Frustration"

Frustration is the only complex emotion that we are equipped with at birth. Of course, we have also been given the ability to experience happiness, sadness, etc. Yet, frustration seems to be more multifaceted, emerging when we realize that the achievability of a goal has been delayed, or obstructed. In infancy, this can be seen with the crying for a bottle. In childhood, this can be seen in temper tantrums for a new toy. As we get older, we must come to realize that this is a terribly inefficient method for achieving our goals. The common theme with the infant wanting the bottle and the child wanting a toy is their reliance on an external source to provide it for them. In learning what a successful person looks like, we have learned that as adults, we must accept responsibility for achieving our own goals, not looking for anyone else to provide it.

This realization, of course, does not provide any relief from frustration. You will sporadically experience frustrations while you are in pursuit of your weight loss goal. A coworker will bring in doughnuts. It will start raining just as you put your walking shoes on. The scale won't budge for a week, even though you have been eating well and exercising. These events can be looked at as minor frustrations that should be easily overcome by using a few tools discussed previously. One that works particularly well is the building of desire. When frustration sets in, reminisce on the desire that catapulted you into your weight loss journey to begin with. Frustrations such as these can cloud the vision of our goal like a dense fog. Think of your goal like a lighthouse. The more you build that desire and concentrate on your goal, the brighter the light will become, and no amount of fog will be able to stop you from reaching your destination.

A more detrimental case of frustration occurs when it is experienced chronically. In this case, there seems to be no reprieve from the frustration. This is often found with one of, or a combination of, two factors. The first factor is having not realized your ability to achieve your realistic goals. We have thoroughly discussed how an unreasonably restricted self-image can impede any goal, so I will leave it at that. The second factor is one of setting unreasonable goals. For example, while it is in your best interest to engage in physical activity if you are trying to lose weight, it is dreadfully unrealistic to set a goal of exercising for two hours every day. Likewise, creating a caloric deficit in your diet will help you burn fat, but setting a goal of five hundred calories a day is terribly unrealistic, not to mention, dangerous. Failure is embedded in these unreasonable goals due to our innate desire for perfection. If your goal is to exercise two hours every day, it is reasonable to fall short and still feel successful. Often with weight loss, the objectives we set for ourselves along the way to our goal, such as exercise, eating more fruits and vegetables, etc., do not have to be met with perfection. If you were to complete most of your workouts and get in most of your servings of fruits and vegetables, the weight loss would come regardless. However, if you view things as a perfectionist, only in black and white, or success and failure, you are likely to find yourself chronically frustrated, and most likely quitting on your goal, and yourself.

"A" is for "Agressiveness"

Think of one of the last times you were frustrated. Maybe you got a flat tire. I bet you slammed the palm of your hand against the steering wheel. Or maybe the grocery bag split open as you carried it to the kitchen. Did you kick the can of peas across the room? Now think about a time you were frustrated with dieting. Let's say your sister surprised you with a birthday cake even though you said you really didn't want one. Could you see yourself getting a little passive-aggressive, rolling your eyes, or being downright mean to her for not listening to you in the first place? Aggression usually follows suit to frustration.

Your goal-striving machinery is much like a steam boiler. You set the goal and fuel the machine, building up energy, in this metaphor, as steam. This steam is necessary for the machine to do its job; however, it can get rather dangerous if there is no safety valve. Many people use exercise as their safety valve, or pressure-release valve, to stop the frustrations of the day from turning into an all-out explosion. Others enjoy painting. Some people cook. Regardless of what it is, it is imperative to have some form of creative expression to release the steam from your boiler. Without this safety valve, the integrity of the entire goal-striving machine is at risk, and the results can be very noticeable. Think of the overworked employee. She already has high blood pressure and ulcers developing. She's been quite rude at work and is always gossiping about her coworkers. As she comes home from work, she stubs her toe, then kicks the cat. This may be a fairly dramatic representation of frustration turning to aggression due to a lack of pressure-release, however, not far from reality in some cases. Aggression includes passive-aggressive behaviors, and those directed at self-destruction. This can be seen in those who eat their way through frustrating times. Unfortunately, this creative release only leads to more anxiety and frustration.

An immense amount of energy is created through the goal-striving process. Channeling that energy through a form of creative release that will collaborate with your goal achievement is only logical. What's your creative release valve?

"I" is for "Insecurity"

Insecurity stems from illogical thinking regarding weight loss. I have intentionally rehashed that commonsensical thinking should lead you to the conclusion that weight loss is possible. Yet, countless times when counseling my clients, I have heard statements such as…

> *"…I just can't exercise as much, or as hard as other people do."*

> *"…I just can't make it to the gym every day."*

> *"…There's no way I will ever reach my goal weight. I still have over one hundred pounds to go!"*

These three statements break three of the cardinal rules in being secure in your abilities to achieve your weight loss goal; respectively, (1) using a false measure, (2) having a perfectionist attitude, and (3) feeling that the problem is too big, or is outside the self-image. Remember these rules when feeling insecure.

1. Never compare yourself to someone else. Only compare yourself to the *you of yesterday*.

2. Losing weight is like playing darts. You don't have hit the bullseye every time to win. You just have to get close. Think in shades of gray, not black and white.

3. If your goal seems too big, break it down into a series of smaller objectives that are more realistic for your current self-image.

"L" is for "Loneliness"

Think back to charity and esteem from the previous Chapter. The process is cyclic. Recognizing the value of others helps you to realize the value of yourself, and vice versa. In my experience, many overweight people have a low self-esteem, often represented by their belief that they contribute much less to a social situation, for instance, than the next person. Research shows that overweight people are more often passed over for promotions at work as well. While it is possible that their employer harbors a stereotype of overweight people, it is also possible that the overweight person acts out in accordance with their low self-esteem, never carrying themselves with the confidence of success. It is easy to fall into your own self-built stereotype regarding overweight people.

"U" is for "Uncertainty"

Elbert Hubbard once said "The greatest mistake a man can make is to be afraid of making one." Uncertainty is the opposite of courage from the success-type personality. This uncertainty can lead to fear of failing or making a mistake, which can then lead to not taking action at all. Keep in mind, perfection is impossible, and our goal-striving servo-mechanism uses negative feedback (lessons learned from failures) to correct the course. However, the course cannot be corrected when you are standing still.

It is not uncommon for people battling uncertainty to look to place blame on external sources. Let me explain with a personal example. I utilize a scale with body composition analyzers with my clients, which can give me insight into not only body weight, but changes in muscle, fat, and hydration levels. Yet, I still have clients that will consistently precede stepping on the scale with a statement such as "My rings are tight, so I may be retaining water." At times, this may very well be true. However, if you are retaining water every time I pull out the scale, you had better go the urologist to get your kidneys checked out. What is most comical and simultaneously tragic about this is my clients know very well that I couldn't care less about what the scale says. I use the scale because my clients expect me to. This leads me to believe they are not giving me an excuse for their failure; they are giving themselves an excuse for their failure.

"R" is for "Resentment"

Resentment is often another means of self-excusal of failure. As much as you should build a desire for success of your goal, you should simultaneously be building a disdain for the lack of success you are currently experiencing. Notice I did not say a disdain for failure. Failures are lessons that can provide valuable insight. Failures are temporary. Learning from a failure is in itself a success. Lack of success can better be defined as standing still, or not taking action. Resentment does not promote action, but just the opposite. It provides a means of making lack of success more palatable.

One might develop resentment for their family that constantly celebrates with food. One might develop resentment for fast food chains making portion sizes unreasonably large. One might develop a personal resentment for years of being overweight taking its toll on the body, making exercise all that more difficult now. Resentment's very nature removes our own control of a situation and places it externally, making us powerless. Lastly, resentment exists in unchangeable past events, making it an irrational behavior.

"E" is for "Emptiness"

If you recall, it is the sole mission of our servo-mechanism to accomplish goals. Accomplishment of these goals can provide us with physical and emotional rewards of a fight well fought and a job well done. A sense of emptiness can set in when we feel as if our goals have been achieved through false pretenses, shortcuts, or cheating. It can leave us with a sense of false accomplishment. Think of a man who has built a small fortune through a lifetime of hard work and labor. There is no doubt that this fortune carries with it a great sense of accomplishment, as he can now provide everything for his family. This man graciously shares his wealth with his son, who quickly becomes a raging alcoholic and drug abuser. You can plug countless celebrity family names into this story. The son's entitlement to a fortune without having to accomplish anything on his own left him feeling empty inside. He then attempted to fill that emptiness with false happiness of drugs and alcohol. Is it so hard to believe that similar things can happen to those of us who turn to weight loss drugs and surgeries? This emptiness ties in with the characteristic of insecurity.

Since the goal is weight loss, one might think that a certain level of success might be yielded from whatever the "quick fix" result is. For example, if you were to have weight loss surgery, such as liposuction, you would have instantaneously reached your goal. If you were to be prescribed prescription medications to suppress your hunger and lose weight, you might reach your goal without effort. However, these methods might provoke that failure characteristic of emptiness. While the surgery or weight loss medications may have helped you reach your goal, it did nothing for how you logically think, emotionally feel, or physically act with food. There can be little sense of accomplishment from achieving a goal through these methods. There was no ground made to expand the self-image. Therefore, the goal of weight loss, even though already achieved, will seem like something that is undeserved. Even worse, you will question your ability to maintain that goal's accomplishment, falling back into previous habits that have been built in to your servo-mechanism over the years.

The Flashing Red Lights of Failure

If you can become familiar with these seven characteristics of the failure-type personality, you can assure yourself that you will experience success. Should you notice yourself embodying one or more of these characteristics, do not panic. Just as a car has indicator lights that alert the driver that something isn't quite right, your mind can be trained to identify these behaviors suited to these characteristics as indicator lights as well. If you were driving to work and your indicator light came on alerting you that you needed windshield wiper fluid, it wouldn't be logical to break down and cry, or leave the car at the scrap yard. You would be aware of the situation and remedy it. If you're internal indicator lights begin to blink, alarming you that you are acting in accordance with one of these seven failure-type characteristics, remedy the situation immediately. This can be done using the following steps:

1. Learning the indicators of the failure-type personality.

2. Recognize the situation for the truth of what it is, not the opinion you are impressing upon it.

3. Taking immediate corrective action to embody an alternate success-type personality characteristic.

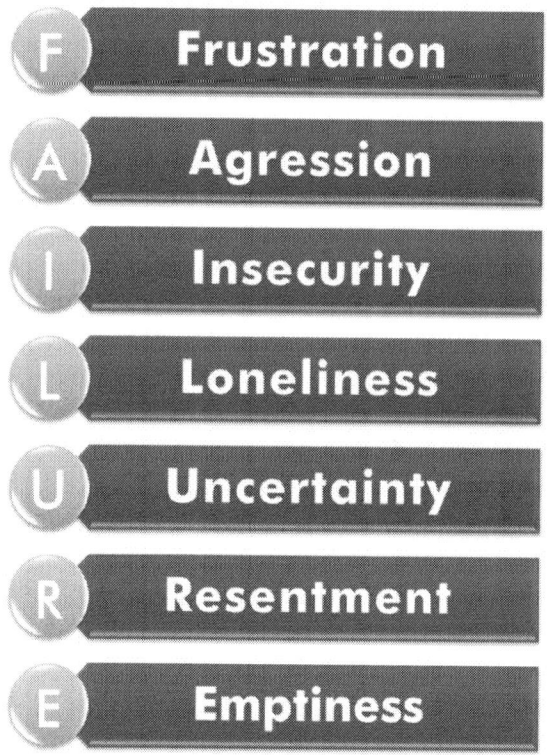

Figure 14. Failure Acronym

Chapter Ten

No Retreat, No Surrender

As the first step into a cold swimming pool is the most difficult, taking the first step towards your weight loss goal is no different. The good news is you have undoubtedly taken your first step towards that goal long ago. Can you even remember the first time you ever tried to lose weight? Me neither. The bad news is once you get out of the cold pool, you will remember just how difficult that first step was the next time you go to take a dip. Again, weight loss is similar. We tend to dwell on the difficulty of the first step when long periods of time lapse in our periodic strides towards our long term goals. Many times this is due to a scarred elf-image.

A Scarred Self-Image

When the physical body is damaged, such as with a cut, the body forms a protective scar. The self-image is similar. It is most likely that the past failures experienced in your struggles with weight loss might have left scars of their own. While physical scars do serve the purpose of protecting you from future attacks, it is likely that you would avoid the behavior that led to the injury, which ultimately left you with that scar. Emotional scars, again, are very similar. It isn't hard to imagine a situation where you have given up on your weight loss goal due to numerous failed attempts. Those failed attempts can cut into your very self-image, making it retreat into a smaller, more protective sphere, as illustrated in Figure 15. Retreating Self-Image.

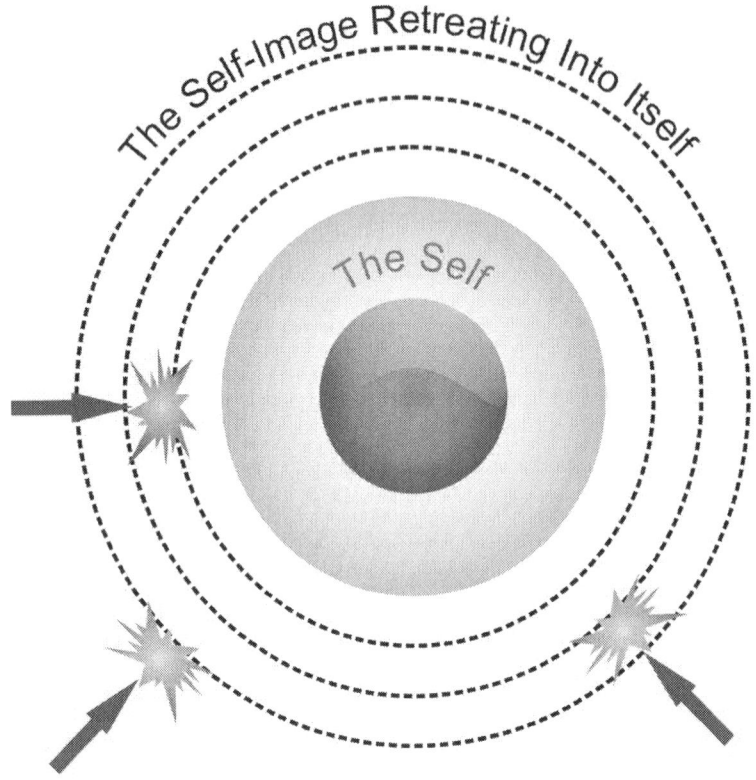

Figure 15. Retreating Self-Image

This shrinking self-image wreaks havoc on your ability to achieve goals, and furthermore, evokes behaviors coinciding with one or more of the failure-type personality characteristics that we have previously addressed. Have you ever said to yourself…

> "…What's the point of trying? I haven't been able to stick to any diet in the past.

> "…There's no point in me joining a gym. I haven't gone for more than a week straight in the past. What makes this time any different?"

> "…Why should I bother even trying to maintain my diet over the holidays? Every party I go to has my favorite cookies. I might as well not even try to fight it."

> "…If my own family doesn't believe I can do it, then why should I?"

Take notice, these statements reflect a situation where you are drawing from your perceptions of past failures that have obviously cut into your self-image, leaving a scar. Worse yet, those scars serve as a reminder that you do not want to experience that failure or embarrassment again. There are two deductions that can be made from events such as these…

> "I make mistakes, but they don't make me. I can learn from the lesson and correct my course."

or

"The humiliation of failure is not worth the risk of trying again."

Remember, the only true failure is the one that stops any further action from happening at all.

Time Heals All Wounds...Slowly

As the old saying goes, "Time heals all wounds." I'm sure that this quote has been repeated millions of times in situations found to be very appropriate. It is also true of the emotional scars inflicted on your self-image when your attempts at losing weight fail. This is demonstrated by the countless times that you have been attempted to lose weight, even after a failure. Let's take a moment to analyze the last time this happened to you. There are two risk factors to look for when multiple attempts at weight loss are being made; (1) the length of time that lapses between attempts at losing weight, more commonly referred to as your "diets", and (2) whether or not you are using the same methods of losing weight that failed you the first time. The very spirit of the statement "time heals all wounds" relies on a passive approach, allowing an excessive amount of time to lapse while the impact of a negative event lessens. This inefficient process can waste valuable time that could have been spent strengthening the self-image by removing the emotional scars. Remember, we said that time can heal wounds, but the scar would remain. This takes us to the second risk factor. If a certain method of trying to lose weight has failed you in the past, why would you try to use it again? Even if that attempt yielded you some progress towards your goal, there is a definitive reason why it did not work. Maybe it was too restrictive of a diet. Maybe the exercise program was too demanding. Maybe you keep bouncing around from one magic pill to the next. Whatever the reason may be, the definition of insanity is doing the same thing over and over while expecting different results.

Fortunately, there are remedies to prevent future emotional scarring, as well as removing old ones.

Preventing Future Scars

While any tool provided within the confines of this text can help to create a strong self-image, there are three specific steps you can take to immunize yourself from the negative consequences of an attack on the self-image; (1) being too big to be threatened, (2) not taking things so personally, and (3) being relaxed.

The first objective should be to achieve a self-image that is so big that an attack on it seems less like a stab wound and more like a mosquito bite. Granted, building a self-image that is that strong will take time and practice of the tools in this book. However, there is a shortcut that you can use in the immediate present the next time you feel your self-image being attacked. You must create a true perception of the situation at hand, and then compare it to a broader span of time. For example, let's say you are in the middle of a successful weight loss endeavor. About eight weeks into this endeavor, your husband surprises you with a weekend getaway. While you are excited that you are taking a little vacation, the first thing that comes to mind is "am I going to be able to stick to my diet and exercise?" You worry if there is a workout room at the hotel. You worry that the portion sizes will be too large. You are worried that any variation from your routine at this point will unravel your progress, and worse yet, lead to regression into old habits. These worrisome thoughts can turn to frustration quite quickly. Now, let's rationally create a true picture of the events at hand. You have been successfully losing weight with your diet and exercise routine for the past eight weeks, almost sixty days. You are going to be taken out of your routine for two days. Even in a worst case scenario, being that there is no workout room at the hotel and the food is less than optimally conducive to weight loss, those two days equal about three percent of the time since you have been successfully losing weight. It is physically impossible to unravel the progress you have made over sixty days in two. The lesson to be learned is your world should not start and stop with each obstacle at hand. In reality, the situation at hand most likely has little bearing on your goals. Being able to identify molehills disguised as mountains indirectly makes your self-image larger by making the attacks on the self-image smaller.

The second objective is to not take everything so personally. Depending on which psychology book you dive in to, you will find that children, sometime within the span of two through seven years of age live in a state of egocentrism. That is to say that they believe that the world revolves around them. It is also said that as age progresses, we will find ourselves growing out of this phase. I would argue that a specific portion of this egocentrism lingers in adulthood. This portion would be the part of us that assumes that, more than not, the negative events in our lives derive from a direct malicious intent from an external source. For example, the snide remarks we absorb at work from the coworker who says "Looks like she's on a diet again" as you pull the salad you brought for lunch out of the employee lounge refrigerator. The truth is, most insensitive remarks have no hidden meaning, and searching for one is a waste of time. The statement your coworker blurted out probably had no malicious intent. Even if it did, its intent most likely manifested from their own frustration of a dilemma that they are going through. That doesn't make it acceptable for people to talk like that to you, but it also does not give you an excuse to let that statement have any effect on your weight loss goals. Simple rational thinking can work your way to that conclusion.

The flipside of this coin of not taking things personally if someone does something to you is not being offended if someone doesn't do something to you. If you have lost weight and are feeling good about yourself, do not feel slighted when your husband doesn't say how nice you look in your new blouse. Do not impose your opinion that he doesn't care. Maybe he doesn't want to imply that you didn't look nice before. Maybe he is just completely ignorant of the fact that you have a new blouse on. Relying on others' recognition of your achievements is a dangerous path, since you are again giving away your control. Humans do have a desire to receive praise and affection, but creating self-reliance for this praise will assure you a consistently strong self-image.

The third objective is to relax. Have you ever noticed how easily your feelings can be hurt when you are suffering the tensions of another negative emotion? Have you ever carried over the frustrations of a bad day at work into your home life? Ever snapped at your child for a rather mediocre situation? The lingering effect of negative emotions triggered from a completely unrelated event is a perfect illustration of how your emotional state can dictate your response to a situation. When you are experiencing a negative emotion, practice consciously identifying it, never letting it carry over to other parts of your life.

Removing Old Scars

The only path to remove old scars is forgiveness. Should someone wrong you, or inflict some type of emotional pain, forgive them, then forget the event. Forgiveness without forgetfulness is pointless. So your coworker made a remark about your salad and you being on a diet again. If you forgive him without forgetting, you will dwell on the event, making much more of it than the actual situation called for. Remember, a majority of hurtful comments are not born from intent, but from what that person is experiencing unrelated to you. If you are not guilty of doing this yourself from time to time, feel free to ignore this lesson. Additionally, if you feel that you have been attacked by someone emotionally, as illustrated by the coworker remarking on your salad, first identify if there is even a reason for your forgiveness. If you come to the conclusion that it is possible that there was no malicious intent driving the comment, there is in fact nothing to forgive. Forgiveness takes practice; first identifying if there is anything to forgive, then forgiving, and then forgetting. The most difficult factor of forgiveness is relinquishing the vindication we experience by "taking the high road." The more frequently you forgive without forgetting can lead to a cycle of seeking out situations where you can assume a martyr's role.

In closing regards to forgiveness, it is imperative that we address forgiving ourselves. It is said that the average person spends upwards of two hours every day feeling guilty about something they have done, or not done. Guilt, remorse, and regret are illogical methods of dealing with situations, as they concentrate on the impossible task of changing past events. Instead of "If I would have only...", try "From now on I will..." Only when you forgive yourself for making mistakes can you learn the lesson and forget the event.

As you very well know, the game of weight loss is vicious, and attackers on your self-image hide around every corner. The only effective way to ward of the attacks is to (1) have a self-image stronger than that of the attacker, (2) not creating an exaggerated perception of an attack by taking events too personally, and (3) forgiving yourself for allowing previous attacks on your self-image to have such long-lasting effects to this point.

Chapter Eleven

Singing in the Rain

Up to this point, you have now learned to identify a host of internal and external obstacles that might stand in the way of your weight loss goals, risking initiation of your failure-type personality. Identifying these obstacles is not enough. You have learned several methods to deal with these obstacles as they arise in your day to day life. Remember, not one of these methods involves avoiding the obstacle altogether. You must embrace the idea that these obstacles exist. There is no magic in this book that will remove obstacles from your path to weight loss glory. However, this book can help you to calmly identify the obstacles, and logically move around them, continuing on your goal's path.

If it is raining outside, would that stop you from going to work? I hope not, and I bet your boss does too. However, this does not mean you shouldn't take precautions from the elements by opening up your umbrella as your step outside. Your umbrella does not stop the rain from falling. You are aware of it, falling all around you. Nonetheless, that umbrella can soften your reaction to the nasty weather.

Think of the rain like the obstacles you will encounter everyday on your pursuit of losing weight, as illustrated in

Figure 16. An Umbrella for Negativity. Just as you cannot make the rain stop falling, it's impossible to stop the obstacles from arising. By learning a few tools presented in this chapter, you can shield yourself from the impact of these obstacles without retreating into the safety of your home.

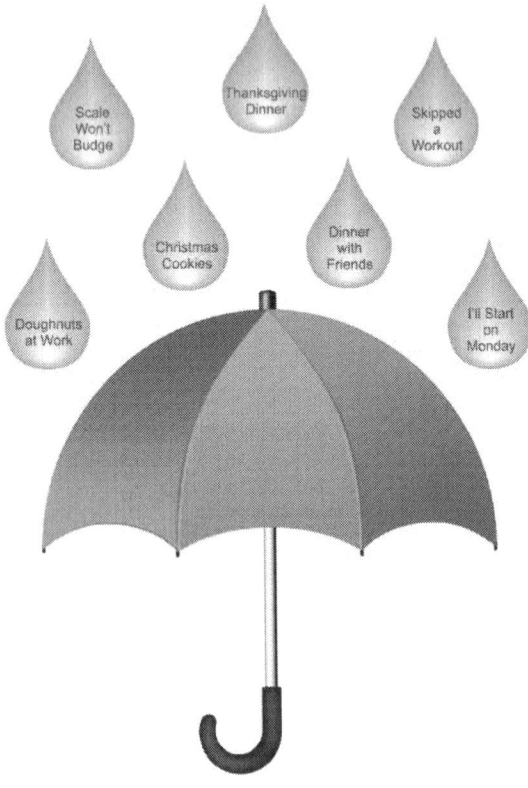

Figure 16. An Umbrella for Negativity

You're Overreacting

It is often not the situation at hand, or decision that needs to be made, that holds great risk. It is often our misinterpretation and drastic overreaction to the situation that gets us into trouble.

In this day and age, mobile phones are less a luxury and more a necessity. A time not long ago, it was perfectly palatable to call someone at home or at work. If that person was unavailable, you would leave a message and your call would be returned at their earliest convenience. A Pandora's Box was opened in the late 1990s, when mobile phones shifted from the hip holsters of lawyers and physicians to the backpacks of children, the pockets of men, and the purses of women. A status quo was established, setting a precedent that at any given time, your family, friends, bosses, coworkers, etc. should be able to get in touch with you on demand. There is a simple solution to this catastrophic condition; turn off your phone, or simply do not answer it.

A normal reaction to a phone call would be to answer it. It takes no conscious thought. If you feel the vibration from your pocket, or as the ringtone hits your ear, you reach for your phone and press talk. Our reactions to everyday stimuli are very similar. Once a situation has presented itself repeatedly, the servo-mechanism takes over and handles the task for us. These are what we call habits. Unfortunately, especially in dealing with body weight, we tend to have several habits that are not so advantageous to our goals.

What is imperative to understand is the fact that just like the phone cannot force you to answer it, the painstaking recurrence of negative stimuli that you endure does not have to responded to out of habit. There are countless instances of our habitual responses to everyday events that lead us down a path of being overweight, for example…

> …you skip breakfast, leading to a deposit of a few dollars to the employee lounge vending machine midmorning.

> …you eat dinner in front of the television, leading to overeating.

> …you eat sweets and chips when you are upset.

> …you automatically postpone your efforts until next Monday when you slip up on your diet or exercise routine.

When it rings, you can refuse to answer your phone. You can also refuse to act out of bad habit.

Act Like a Man

In the late nineteenth century, a scientist named Ivan Pavlov studied the topic of classic conditioning, meaning programmed responses, or habit. In his famous study, Pavlov would introduce food to a dog to generate a response of salivation. This was a natural, instinctual response. He then would introduce the food to the dog, while simultaneously ringing a bell. The dog would continue to salivate when the food was presented. Pavlov then noticed that when he rang the bell, the dog would begin to salivate, even without the presentation of food. This dog had been "conditioned" to believe that when the bell rang, food would be presented. The dog was salivating out of habit, as there was no other reason for a bell to make a dog salivate.

This is how all of our habits, both good and bad, manifest. We learn to react in a certain way to a condition, and soon enough that reaction becomes second nature, a product of the servo-mechanism at work. Regarding Pavlov's experiment, the conditioned response of salivation would eventually subside if the bell ringing was not reinforced with presentation of food. In a sense, the dog unlearned the conditioned response. Here is an optimistic piece of information. Dogs do not have the creative mechanisms that humans have. While a dog would require a certain amount of time to pass without the introduction of the stimuli to overcome a bad habit, human beings possess the ability to utilize our rational thought, creative imagination, and will to stop an automatic reaction from occurring. Quintessentially, humans do not have to "answer the phone". By identifying an unhealthy habit, a human being can effectively stop the reaction from happening, using creative imagination to determine an alternative reaction that is healthier, and impose exertion, or will, to make that new reaction take place. Over time, this new reaction will replace the former bad habit.

There will be instances when you will be unable to put off making a decision indefinitely. As I mentioned earlier, it is a common reaction to suspend your healthy efforts until next Monday when a slipup occurs. Many people immediately decide that, for some mystic reason, next Monday will yield better results, leading to overconsumption for the several days leading to next week. The next time you experience a small misstep in your routine, delay making a hasty decision by jumping off the deep end into a pool of potato chips. Simply tell yourself "I do not have to make my decision now." Much like pressing the snooze button on your alarm clock, or sending a call to voice mail, you can get to making that decision later, when there is less emotional interference to worry about. By consciously and forcefully dictating a delay in response, you can disrupt the normal habitual or programmed response, allowing you to creatively reprogram yourself to institute a new, healthier habit.

Build Yourself a Happy Place

As I briefly touched upon previously, there is no worse time to make a decision than when your emotional state is negatively exaggerated in any way. One way to cope would be to wait until the negative emotional state passes, making your decision in a rational state of mind. We can also expedite this process by using our "Theater of the Mind" trick introduced several Chapters ago. If you recall, the physical body will experience emotions correlative to what the brain is experiencing. If you are rehashing an infuriating moment in your mind from a past event, you would experience the same anger as if it just happened, given that your imagination's recollection of the situation was vivid enough. However, this would not be a good state of mind to make a rational decision. It is easy to be overcome by negative emotions, having them influence your subsequent reaction. On the other hand, if you can evoke a sense of relaxation through a corresponding vivid image, you can rest assured that your next reaction will be of sound derivation.

If you have been practicing utilizing your mind's theater from Chapter Three, you should be well equipped to implement this next tool. The objective is to create a place where nothing can bother you, a sanctuary, if you will. Make this place as brilliantly detailed as possible. It may take time. Rome wasn't built in a day. There are no rules or regulations as to what your sanctuary has to offer. You can choose the structure, the colors, the interior attributes, even what the exterior looks like as you approach your destination. To start, retreat here once a day, or a few times per week, each time including more and more details that will only add to the pleasantness and relaxation of your visit. Through time and repetition, you will find that your sanctuary can be instantaneously accessed through your creative imagination, leaving you feeling nothing but pure respite from your worries. The better you can become at creating, and more repetitiously you visit your sanctuary, the more secure you can feel that your subsequent decisions and reactions will be of reliable origin, without the infringement of negative emotions.

Cleansing Your Emotional Palate

Using your mind's theater to create a sanctuary from negative emotions is one of the most effective tools that Dr. Maltz provided. However, some people may feel silly attempting to create a vacation home in their mind. Luckily, there are other ways to achieve this type of emotional clarity.

Negative emotions can linger long after the causative situation has passed, much like a strong flavor can linger in the mouth long after the food was eaten. I'm sure your kids would agree after the reaction they received following asking you for a ride to the mall after you just got home from an exhausting and frustrating day at work. Again, the first step is to identify that you are experiencing a negative emotion, or have reacted or overreacted uncharacteristically to unrelated situation due to that negative emotion. Once recognized, picture yourself swishing around some emotional mouthwash, then spitting it out, along with all the negative emotions. Repeat this process until you can diagnose that there are no lingering negative emotions.

Just like running ten programs on your computer simultaneously, your servo-mechanism can become overwhelmed and confused if you are attempting to make positive decisions while experiencing negative emotions.

Chapter Twelve

Under Pressure

Sink or swim. This is an idiom commonly used to suggest that one has but two choices; overcome the obstacle at hand and succeed, or be overcome by the obstacle and fail, mainly pertaining to one's own competence and diligence. Less commonly known, this saying is thought to originate from early barbaric practices of placing weights on an alleged witch and submerging her in water. Should the accused manage to stay afloat, they were determined to be in contract with the devil and subsequently executed. If they were to drown, they were exonerated of all charges. This is a clear example of a poor way to obtain information. Peculiarly enough, the most literal interpretation of this saying is also a quite poor way of learning a new skill.

What is the best way to learn how to swim? One thing is for sure. Being tossed into the deep end is not the answer. In fact, the process of learning any new skill cannot be done efficiently while under the influence of elevated pressure. Neuroscience can explain how while learning a new skill set, the brain will create a mental map that can be accessed when confronted with a similar situation in the future. When experienced in a non-threatening, unexcited environment, these mental maps are broad. A broad mental map allows for the application of this knowledge to other related activities. When experienced in a pressurized, over-motivating environment, these mental maps become narrow. A narrow mental map reduces the ability to apply these skills to similar circumstances. Therefore, if you were to be thrown in to a deep swimming pool with no previous experience or swimming skills, a narrow mental map would be formed on how to stay afloat in a crude fashion, based on survival instinct alone. Should you be eased into a shallow swimming pool with proper instruction of how to coordinate muscle movements to glide through the water, all with the security that should you begin to sink, you could simply place your feet on the bottom and stand upright, a broad mental map would form.

This concept is further supported with the example of a mouse and a maze. In a controlled environment, if a mouse is allowed to freely explore the maze, once finding the exit, the mouse will effectively learn, or remember the route, and be able to repeat it. This process appears to work even better when a reward, such as food, is placed at the end of the maze. When the same mouse is put into a state of starvation, the results become less efficient. The mouse will eventually find the exit to the maze, however, the ability to reproduce the results declines significantly. By creating a situation that is overly motivating, the ability to learn and remember the skill suffers.

Think of a time when you were caught off guard by someone tossing a mean-spirited comment your way. You sit there and stare, as if a mute, only to have dozens of witty comebacks come to mind after that person has left the room. All of these examples, from swimming, to the maze, to a simple comeback have one thing in common. They identify that the conscious mind cannot utilize the creative process to solve a problem when overly motivated in a pressure situation. In moments such as this, it is the job of the servo-mechanism to step in and react. If not well prepared, the servo-mechanism's reaction may be less than satisfactory. This Chapter will identify several methods of handling the high-stress situations that gravitate, often in the most inopportune times, towards those attempting to lose weight.

Becoming a Weight Loss Natural

We all know someone who is very good at what they do. A salesperson that is handed the assignment when a major account is on the line. An athlete who the coach wants to get the ball to when the game is on the line. Someone who is *clutch*, or *a natural*.

Ponder for a moment the essence of the moniker *natural*, or the phrase "It comes naturally to them." If you have been welcoming the lessons of this book into your mind, you might come to the conclusion that if someone is doing something that comes naturally to them, they are in fact acting out in accordance with the servo-mechanism. After all, the servo-mechanism simply strives towards your goal, assuming your goal is harmonious with your self-image. As we have previously discussed, the self-image is not static, rather a dynamic facet of the personality that can be shaped and molded, either positively or negatively. People who are referred to as *clutch* have undoubtedly shaped their self-image to be able to allow goals to be established and acted upon without foreseeing obstacles as points of defeat. These success-oriented traits are not reserved for a select few. These traits are available to all of us. This is not a discussion about talent. While an individual's *talent* is a wonderful catalyst of success, anyone can develop the *skills* necessary to turn an obstacle into success, or a crisis into opportunity. In fact, the very word *crisis* is derived from the Greek word meaning decisiveness, or point of decision.

It is easy to visualize a "natural" in the form of an athlete. They have a unique skill set that affords them the ability to perform well during high-stress points of opportunity. But can a person become a natural at losing weight? To be honest, this task is much easier than that of an athlete.

Practice Makes Perfect

Most of us have encountered a situation that resembles that of a crisis, or a situation where that next act carries with it an inflated amount of importance. A presentation to your coworkers, perhaps; or giving a toast at your best friend's wedding. What about a situation regarding your health or body weight? It may be more difficult to find an example such as this, yet, every decision made regarding your body weight seems to have this type of impending consequence...

"... What will I order tonight when we go out to eat?"

"...Will I have the motivation to go on my walk tonight?"

"...What will they have to eat at this party?"

For now, let's just assume that you are justified in thinking that these events, and your approach to handling them, have a greater consequence than usual. How do you prepare? I am well known by my clients for answering questions with questions; so I may retort "How does an athlete prepare?" It is impossible for an athlete to practice in situations of game-changing orientation. A baseball player cannot actually create a situation where there are two outs in the ninth inning, and they are up to bat. But what the ball player can do is practice in an environment that is not overly stimulating. The ball player can take hundreds of swings at batting practice, getting to know how every single pitch might look as it approaches home plate, how to make contact with that pitch, and how to place the hit where desired. You can do this as well. In fact, you already do. Every moment of every day you are making decisions that translate into whether or not you are losing or gaining weight. If you are actively attempting to live a lifestyle based in healthy habits, then you have been practicing for these crises all along. So...

"... What will I order tonight when we go out to eat?"

"Why am I even worried about it? I have been there numerous times. I know they serve healthy options. I'll just make sure to have a small snack before we go so I can avoid the basket of bread and ordering any appetizers."

"...Will I have the motivation to go on my walk tonight?"

"Of course I will. I am exhausted every day after work, and today will be no different. I have been able to go walking after much harder days of work than this."

"...What will they have to eat at this party tonight?"

"I suppose it doesn't matter. I cannot control what they serve me. What I can control is how much of it I actually eat. I have been monitoring my portions for weeks now and am confident that I can do the same there. I have taught myself not to pick at things throughout the day, so that will not serve as a problem this evening either."

You have developed a skill set of behaviors that will facilitate you losing weight. You have practiced these behaviors consistently since you began your last weight loss attempt. You have become good at acting out those behaviors. When the game is on the line, you already know what to do.

The Best Defense is a Good Offense

A motto commonly heard in football locker rooms is "the best defense is a good offense." So what does that mean? In regards to the sport of football, it essentially suggests that the best way to keep the opponent from scoring points is to keep the ball in your team's possession. It may sound comical; however, the game of weight loss can be approached in this same manner.

If you have effectively devised a goal and communicated that goal with your servo-mechanism, then you are on offense. You have the ball. You are in control of every decision that you make. This does not mean that the opposition is going to lie down as you progress to your goal. There will be obstacles that appear to be attempting to prevent you from obtaining success, just as a defense attempts to prevent the offense from scoring. It is important to take an aggressive stance, rather than defensive. A passive, defensive approach to weight loss insinuates that you are standing your ground in the face of an adverse situation, however, not moving forward. An aggressive attitude will assure all actions are deriving from your desire to progress towards your goal, overcoming all obstacles placed in front of you. An example seems fitting here. Imagine you find yourself a few weeks in to your latest attempt to achieve a healthy weight, when adversity arises. You are going on vacation with your family. While this is undoubtedly an event that is delighting, you can't help but worry about what is going to happen to the healthy behaviors you have adopted recently. A passive, defensive approach to this might sound like…

> "…I'm going to allow myself to have some fun on vacation. I will allow myself to eat desserts, but will try to watch everything else. I won't worry about exercising since we will be walking quite a bit."

Please, do not feel slighted if this previous response is something you can visualize yourself saying. It is neither incorrect, nor correct. However, it is passive and defensive. In this example, you find yourself absorbing the impact of the obstacles arising around you. You are attempting to minimize the damage, or the retreat, but you are not progressing forward. With a more aggressive stance, it might sound more like…

> "…Just because I am on vacation does not mean I have to abandon my healthy habits. Eating desserts will not add enjoyment to my vacation. The hotel we are staying at has a gym, so I can hop on the treadmill for a half hour every day before my family even gets out of bed."

In this response, you should be able to hear the tone difference. There is nothing passive about your stance here. You have decided to continue to enact your healthy behaviors, and have planned to proceed actively towards your goal.

Weight loss can be a grueling process. At times, it will seem like all you can handle to simply stand your ground. However, the more often that you can find yourself acting and reacting in an aggressive manner, the more efficient you will be at achieving your goal.

Not Every Moment is "Do or Die"

Bases loaded with two outs in the ninth.

Down by one and shooting free throws with no time left on the clock.

Trailing by two and a forthcoming field goal attempt with time expiring.

Leading by two strokes on the eighteenth hole with a ten foot putt decisively standing between winning and losing, success and failure.

The common denominator of these situations, the very spirit that defines clutch athletes, is that they are able to perform at their highest level when placed in a situation that has inflated importance, and therefore, exacerbated stress. If applying logical thinking, the skills needed to complete the task should not be affected by the situation. The baseball player who steps to the plate with the bases loaded and two outs should have the same probability of a successful outcome that they always have. If their batting average is .333, they should have a thirty three percent chance of getting a hit. If the basketball player who is awarded two free throw attempts at the end of a game after being fouled just as time expires usually makes ninety percent of his free throws, there is a very good chance of him making those next two. The golfer staring at a ten foot putt to win should have made this shot several times in the past. Yet, the external influences of the situation, such as the game being on the line, do have drastic impact on an athlete's performance. It is their ability, or inability to perform at that moment that will be remembered, thus defining if they are a clutch player.

Here is the good news. There is absolutely no such instance in your life that will ever hold the same over-inflated importance as one of these situations. By no means do I intend to infer that decisions you make regarding your health, diet, and exercise are any less important than that of a sporting event. What I am intending to convey is that these decisions you make on a day to day, moment to moment basis, are countless in number. Regarding the golf example, and for those of you who do not know the game, a *mulligan*, as defined by Merriam Webster, is "a free shot sometimes given a golfer in informal play when the previous shot was poorly played". Every decision you make regarding your health comes with unlimited mulligans! This is what we have referred to throughout the book as immediate course correction. If you were to decide at this moment to put down this book, pick up a doughnut and devour it, I would identify that as missing your putt. If you were to convince yourself that you do not want to go to the health club tonight, I would identify that as missing your putt. If you were to decide to all together abandon your healthy behaviors while on vacation, I would identify that as missing your putt. So take your mulligan! No, you cannot take back these moments in time, and any effort spent doing so is pointless. Remember, attempting to change the past is illogical and will provide no use. However, you can course correct and get it right at every subsequent opportunity.

One unfortunate attribute of the majority of people attempting to lose weight is the uncanny ability to make every single moment in their lives pertaining to their weight a crisis event. Every single moment seems to be misconstrued to have some life-altering consequence, impressing a level of utmost importance, and subsequent amplified stress. Of course, this level of stress, even for the clutch player, can negatively impact the result. So it is up to you. Would you rather live in a world where every moment and every decision carries with it the pressure of a "do or die" situation? Or would you rather live in a world where every shot you take has unlimited "do-overs?" No one else is enforcing your perception that you either have to eat perfect while on vacation or you have to act gluttonous. You are the one creating the situation around the decision. It lies in your creative imagination. The choice is yours.

Chapter Thirteen

In Summary

If you have read this book from start to finish, I applaud your efforts. As weight loss is a journey, so too is the progression of this text. We started with a few simple ideas, expounded upon them in repetitious, and sometimes grueling fashion. At very least I hope that at times, you were greeted with "Aha!" moments of clarity; and during some of those times, I am sure these moments were not as welcome as others. In researching the premise of this book, I found that truth is sometimes a bitter pill to swallow; that same truth that we spend so much time seeking about the secret of successful weight loss can be hard to confront when staring it in the eyes. This can be especially true if you have come to the realization, as I have, that deceptive weight loss product marketing, "super-sized" fast food value meals, or simple genetics are *not* the obstacles needed to be overcome in your pursuit of a healthy body.

In the Beginning

As I have stated throughout this book, I cannot take credit for the science that it is based upon. While pulling information from famous scholars and philosophers, the primary foundation of this book is based upon the work of

Dr. Maxwell Maltz. Dr. Maltz, a plastic surgeon, began his practice in the 1920s. Through decades of practice, and spurred by an ever-increasing traffic of patients searching to better themselves through plastic surgery, Maltz became progressively spellbound by (1) the number of those patients who possessed a radically overstated mental visualization of their physical ailment, and (2) those patients who continued to hold on to their insecurities even after the surgery had been completed, leaving a physical resemblance of perfection.

In 1960 Maltz published his first compilation of ideas as a new science of self-help, a science he referred to as Psycho-Cybernetics. Since then, Dan Kennedy, with the help of Dr. Maltz' wife and The Psycho-Cybernetics Foundation, has expounded the science, initiating a renaissance for ideas that helped millions of people realize their true potential. Taken directly from the pages of *THE NEW PSYCHO-CYBERNETICS*,

> *"The essence of Psycho-Cybernetics is the accurate, calm, and ultimately automatic separation of fact from fiction, fact from opinion, actual circumstance from magnified obstacle, so that our actions and reactions are solidly based on truth, not our own or others' opinions."*

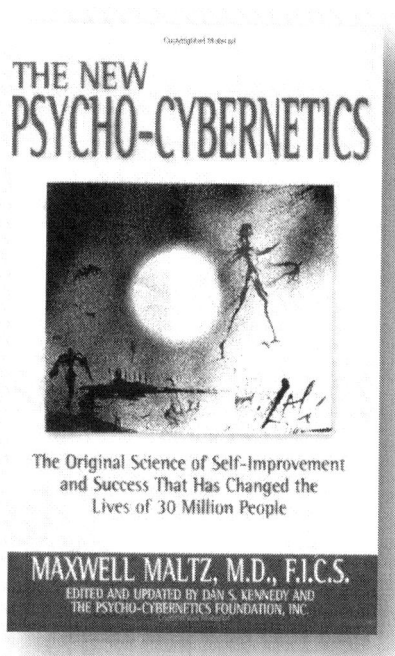

Figure 17. THE NEW PSYCHO-CYBERNETICS

But what exactly is the science of psycho-cybernetics?   As
Maltz would explain,

> *You might think of Psycho-Cybernetics as a*
> *collection of insights, principles, and practical*
> *methods that enable you to do all of the following:*

> 1. *Conduct an accurate inventory and analysis of*
>   *the contents of your self-image.*
> 2. *Identify   erroneous   and   restrictive*
>   *programming imbedded in your self-image and*

systematically alter it to better suit your purposes.

3. *Use your imagination to reprogram and manage your self-image.*

4. *Use your imagination in concert with your self-image to effectively communicate with your servo-mechanism, so that it acts as an Automatic Success Mechanism, moving you steadily toward your goals, including getting back on course when confronted with obstacles.*

5. *Effectively use your servo-mechanism as something like a giant search engine, to provide precisely the idea, information, or solution you need for any particular purpose – even reaching beyond your own stored data to obtain it.*

In a way, Psycho-Cybernetics is a communication system, for effectively communicating with yourself.

Zero Resistance Weight Loss is an original work, based on THE original self-improvement science. Down to the title, this book is a tribute to the vast applications that Psycho-Cybernetics can reach; the title *Zero Resistance Weight Loss* is a play on one of Dr. Maltz' other works, *Zero Resistance Selling*, a book designed to apply the principles of Psycho-Cybernetics to the sales profession. The subtitle of this book, *How To Lose Weight Naturally And Fast,* is not at all meant to be misleading. There is no more a natural way to lose weight than to seek to do so through Psycho-Cybernetics, and there is no faster way to accomplish this task than being able to course correct immediately after every misstep, a key to this science. Again, I do not take credit for the science encompassed in this text. I recognize Dr. Maltz for the pioneer that he was, and thank him for the gift that he has given us. I implore you to seek out a copy of Psycho-Cybernetics. You will find that I have not attempted to change the concepts at all, only concentrate their applications. I simply have taken the concepts and modified them to more concisely apply them to losing weight. I have found it my calling to take this science and apply it to the field that I have spent my life studying. After all, what better way to illuminate the shortcomings of the field of weight loss than attacking, head on, the main obstacle most, if not all of us share in our attempts at slim body...ourselves.

In Review

Let's take a look back at what you have learned thus far. Think of this section as a review, and your road map to success. I encourage you to read this book as often as needed; but when you have a certain topic you want to refresh yourself on, this would be the place to start.

Chapter One Core Elements

The self-image acts as a filter between what your conscious mind wants and what your subconscious mind will strive for. This self-image is built through your past experiences, both good and bad. This process of constructing the self-image is called imprinting, the degree of which your past experiences play a role being dictated by three factors; (1) authoritative source of the event, (2) intensity at which you experienced it, and (3) repetition of experiencing similar events and outcomes. While it is the function of your conscious mind to facilitate a goal, such as weight loss, your subconscious mind, or servo-mechanism, may never receive that goal if it is inconsistent with your current self-image.

Chapter Two Core Elements

In expanding on the idea of your subconscious mind, or servo-mechanism, it essentially is a guidance system, or goal-striving machine that can be programmed to complete a vast majority of the work needed to accomplish you goal. To engage this powerful tool, you must (1) choose your goal, (2) take action to progress towards that goal, (3) make errors, and (4) effectively and efficiently correct those errors. This entire process is dependent on the fact that you will make mistakes; however, you will correct those mistakes in expedited fashion. This process can be seen at work in everyday arbitrary examples such as tying your shoes, or driving to work. Any task that is completed mostly without conscious effort is an example of your servo-mechanism at work.

Your servo-mechanism is a servant of the goals that you implement, and is limited only by your self-image. If your self-image does not accept the pending outcome of the goal you set, you will not be able to process that work order to your servo-mechanism. It is your self-image that dictates whether your servo-mechanism will function as your automatic success or your automatic failure mechanism.

Chapter Three Core Elements

Your imagination is a formidable ally on your path to success. Hypnosis, a potent form of imagination, is proof of this. Research has concluded that should a person believe what they are experiencing in their mind, then the body will react in that way. A rather negative illustration of this can be found in the life of an anorectic, a person held hostage by the vivid false belief, or illusion of being overweight, although all physical truths indicate otherwise.

On a more positive note, this same powerful tool, your imagination, can be used in a much more constructive manner. As seen with the anorectic, the physical body cannot distinguish between reality and vivid imagination or perception. This can also be seen by someone who is convinced, or hypnotized, that they are cold and will experience goose bumps, even though the actual environment is quite temperate. You can create any story that you wish to experience those respective physiologic responses and emotions, similar to that of the emotions you experience when watching your favorite "feel god" movie; except this movie will be viewed in your mind. Make this movie as elaborate as possible, including detail after detail, visualizing yourself experiencing the utmost success in accomplishing your goal. Practice this until you can physically feel the emotion that would accompany this success, as if it had already happened.

Chapter Four Core Elements

To effectively change, or dehypnotize yourself, you must (1) identify the false perception, (2) challenge this false perception, and (3) replace this false perception with the truth. There is little doubt that you maintain some sort of negative hypnotic state today. For example, you might truly believe, either consciously or subconsciously, that you do not have the ability to lose weight, a false perception that has been fortified by negative imprinting. This false perception must be uprooted prior to setting a goal of weight loss and taking action. Otherwise, you will find yourself operating against your self-image under sheer willpower, ultimately leading to failure, or "snap-back."

A fundamental component of successful goal accomplishment is establishing a true self-image; not one of deflated or inflated perception. A deflated perception, also known as an inferiority complex, is often seen through the act of false measure; or comparing your abilities to that of someone else. An inflated perception, also known as a superiority complex, in most cases is seen in people that secretly harbor an inferiority complex. The superiority complex acts as a shield, or defense mechanism, in attempt to hide their own insecurities; a trait embodied by the stereotypical schoolyard bully.

Chapter Five Core Elements

The power of the conscious mind pales in comparison the capabilities of the subconscious servo-mechanism in regards to goal accomplishment. However the conscious mind is invaluable concerning your ability to mold your self-image, allowing you unlimited growth potential. Your self-image cannot be changed by willpower, but it can be changed by realizing the truth of a situation, rather than the false perceptions you harbor. This can be accomplished by asking yourself the following series of questions:

1. *Why   do   I   believe   I   can't*
    _____?
2. *Is this belief based on actual fact or on an assumption?*
3. *Is there any rational reason for such a belief?*
4. *Is it possible that I am mistaken in thinking this?*
5. *Would I come to the same conclusion about someone else in a similar situation?*
6. *Why should I continue to act and feel as if this were true if there is no good reason to believe it?*

Often times, a negative self-image, or false perception of yourself is the result of your interpretation of past events; however, there is no need to rehash these past events. In fact, reliving a negative moment from your past can evoke those same negative emotions you were feeling at the time of the event. Instead, think of the past like digging for gold. Take with you the lesson that can be learned from the event, such as why you might have failed, and what you can do to course correct in the future, and leave the rest behind, in essence, taking with you what's valuable, and leaving behind the worthless weight.

Chapter Six Core Elements

Weight loss requires a certain skill set, like any other goal worth accomplishing. Acquiring this skill set requires progression through four phases of learning:

1. *Unconscious Incompetence: characterized by not knowing if you have a certain skill, simply because you have never tried.*

2. *Conscious Incompetence: usually initiated once a new goal is set. This phase is characterized by struggle in progressing towards a goal, as the conscious mind is responsible for the work.*

3. *Conscious Competence: as time progresses and you continue to action towards your goal, your skill set develops. Effort is still being applied; however, a portion of the workload is shifted to the servo-mechanism.*

4. *Unconscious Competence: the final stage of the learning process. This phase is characterized by a complete development of a skill set, so fined tune that conscious effort is no longer*

needed. The behaviors that engage those skills are driven by habit, deriving from the servo-mechanism.

There are a few ways to expedite this learning process. First, once a goal is set, no time should be spent second guessing it. Similar to roulette, you have placed your bet and the wheel is spinning. It is futile to worry about the negative at this point. Second, focus on the here and now, concentrating your efforts in the moment. The past is unchangeable and the future unpredictable; however, the actions you engage in now will shape your future to yield what you desire. Third, prioritize your tasks, and the handling of your goal's obstacles, by the level of detriment they pose in negating your efforts. The opposite of this would be procrastination, a goal killer.

Chapter Seven Core Elements

While any goal with a foreseeable positive outcome is good, one that is vague in nature can impair the best of efforts. A well-developed goal can make your progression towards success that much easier. To assure a well-developed, or *SMART* goal, it must meet five specific criteria; (1) specific, (2) measurable, (3) attainable, (4) relevant, and (5) time-sensitive.

With your goal now being well-developed, progressing towards it should be accompanied by a level of happiness. Vice versa, a level of happiness can catalyze your progression towards your goal. In this cycle, it does not matter which comes first, the happiness or the success, as both will breed each other. To remain in this cycle, there are a handful of pitfalls that should be avoided that can gravitate you towards unhappiness and failure:

1. Being Happy Being Unhappy: often seen as a characteristic of people who find a warped sense of contentment doing for others instead of for themselves, out of desire for attention of their sacrifice. This is commonly referred to as "playing the martyr-role".

2. Looking Forward to Happiness: often seen as a characteristic of those who think in terms of black and white, such as only being happy once the ultimate goal is achieved, but experiencing no happiness that comes for the series of accomplishments on the path to achieving their goal.

3. Taking Things Personally: often seen as a characteristic of people who feel like every obstacle they encounter on their path was specifically designed for them. Most often, these arbitrary annoyances have no personal intent of impeding progress.

4. Imparting Opinion in Lieu of Fact: built on taking things too personally, these people may also imply their own negative opinion to an arbitrary event, such as believing someone is talking about

you, simply because they glanced at you during their conversation with someone else.

The first step to remaining in the happiness-success cycle is to be able to identify these negative behaviors in yourself. Once you begin the recognition process, immediately block the thought from turning into action by developing a mantra that will eliminate the negative consequence. An example of this might be mentally picturing yourself "X'ing Out" of an annoying popup while you are on your computer. If you are to practice this with intent, the intervention will become habit, and effortless.

Chapter Eight Core Elements

There are seven unique characteristics often found in those people who effortlessly find success. Those characteristics can easily be remembered with the acronym *SUCCESS*.

Sense of Direction: having a goal.

Understanding: searching for, and comprehending the knowledge of what is needed to reach that goal.

Courage: the drive to put that knowledge into action, even if temporary failure is imminent.

Charity: believing in the worth of all people, and their right to be treated with respect.

Esteem: believing in the worth of yourself, and your right to be treated with respect.

Self-Confidence: believing that just as every minor failure in your past has chipped away at your self-image, even the smallest success can help to build it.

Self-Acceptance: understanding that you cannot manifest any special powers through the practice of these methods, but that you already have these abilities which are only being hindered by your insufficient self-image.

Chapter Nine Core Elements

Just as successful people share common characteristics, those who repeatedly invite failure have similar traits as well, spelled out in the acronym *FAILURE*.

Frustration: feeling helpless to the obstacles presenting themselves around you.

Aggressiveness: often spawned through frustration, expelling pent up creative energy in noncreative ways.

Insecurity: found in false perceptions, feeling that you do not possess the ability to overcome an obstacle.

Loneliness: in cyclic fashion, believing you have less to offer than someone else, causing you to retreat into solitude.

Uncertainty: a paralyzing fear of making a mistake, even though logical thinking tells you more progress can be made from correcting a mistake than not making one at all.

Resentment: a mask for its true name; jealousy. Feeling victimized by nature in comparison to others' successes.

Emptiness: a lack of happiness from accomplishing a goal while believing that accomplishment was not warranted by your actions.

Learning to identify these characteristics in your behaviors can act as warning indicators, signifying a need to correct your behavioral course and redirect to success-type behaviors.

Chapter Ten Core Elements

As the physical body incurs injury, a protective scar is formed to prevent further damage to that area in the future. Unfortunately, the self-image has the same defense mechanism that acts as a barrier, not allowing you to experience events that will strengthen and expand the self-image. A valuable skill set to develop is how to prevent new scars from forming, as well as how to remove the existing emotional scars.

Preventing new emotional scars can be accomplished in three easy steps.

1. Be Too Big to be Threatened

    Avoid the overreaction to an obstacle, or a temporary failure. Many times we react to adversity as if we have been stabbed by a sword, rather than pricked by a pin. By strengthening the self-image, you can make yourself much bigger than the looming threat.

2. Don't Take Things So Personally

    When confronted by an insensitive remark or gesture, a weak self-image can be bruised quite easily. Removing the personal nature of such an attack can lessen the injury. Most insensitive remarks and action of others directed towards you have no personal intent, rather they have manifested from the other person's own internal struggle of a weak self-image.

3. Relax

    Negative aggressiveness is often caused by elevated frustration. The emotions that circle this frustration can taint all subsequent action, such as taking out the emotions of an unrelated event on someone else. Relaxation exercises and rational thinking can eliminate this unwarranted negativity.

Removing old scars holds separate challenges. However challenging, the process only involves two steps.

1.   Forgive Others, and Forget

Forgiveness of others, at times, can be difficult.   Nonetheless, it is imperative in pursuit of your goal. If you perceive that someone has wronged you, remember to apply rational thinking in attempt to not take such events too personally. If you recall, most times that we feel attacked, there was actually no mal-intent from the offending party; rather, we experienced an action that was a consequence of that person's life. If you can come to this realization, that no intent was behind you being harmed, you will realize there is actually no act to forgive. And then forget.   Without   forgetting,   you   are condemned to rehash the past. Take with it the lesson, and leave behind them burden.

2.   Forgive Yourself

Should you possess the characteristics of a failure-type personality, you may again find yourself rehashing past failures. This action is illogical, and has no place in your life. You make mistakes, but they do not make you. The mistakes simply serve as lessons to be learned from. Learning to forgive yourself for past failures is essential to progressing towards your goal.

Chapter Eleven Core Elements

There are times when not acting will actually be more beneficial that acting hastily. This non-action is warranted when attempting to break bad habits. Throughout your life, you have developed automatic reactions that will yield results contradictory to your goal. For example, you might decide to not exercise one afternoon after feeling guilty about a large lunch. The second step of removing a bad habit is replacing it with a more productive one. Yet, this second step cannot be engaged until you first learn to recognize the bad habit and stop, or at least delay the reaction.

Three concepts can be implemented in attempt to halt or delay an automatic undesirable habit.

1. While humans are "creatures of habit", you do possess the gift of free will. By identifying this trait, you can make a

logical assessment that the habit does not
need to continue.

2. To reduce the frustration of experiencing a
    bad habit, you must develop skills that
    will help you relax. An effective method
    of relaxation is to create a vivid mental
    picture that will evoke positive emotions.
    Utilize the theater of your mind.

3. Do not allow any negative emotions you
    are experiencing to dictate your response
    to unrelated events. Cleanse your palate
    of these negative emotions.

After using these tools to identify negative habits, you can
effectively learn to block them before they manifest. Here
lays your prime opportunity to replace that behavior with a
new, healthy habit.

Chapter Twelve Core Elements

After effectively learning to identify a habitual action that
yields a negative consequence, you will have to employ
effort and will to stop that behavior and implement a new
one. And just as that negative behavior, repeated over time,
developed into a habit, a new behavior that is imposed
willfully and repetitively will become a habitual response.

1. Make it a point to implement the same
    new behavior when you would normally
    perform the negative habit. An example

would be taking a walk when you get home from work when you have noticed you normally go straight to the pantry to grab a bag of chips.

2. Once the new behavior has been established, learn to react to this situation aggressively. Do not simply avoid going to the pantry. Aggressively substitute your new behavior of walking.

3. Don't take yourself too seriously. Not every moment you encounter carries with it the weight of the world. Should you make the mistake of finding yourself holding the bag of chips on the couch, and not out walking around the block, do not assume your bad habit is back. It was a simple mistake that can be undone at the moment of recognition.

In the Zone

I am certain that at this point, if you have embraced the core concepts of this book and implemented its lessons, you are at a pinnacle of weight loss success that you never previously dreamed possible. Additionally, I am hopeful and confident that your success is coming faster and easier than ever. That feeling that you have brewing inside you…that's what Maltz would call "that winning feeling." Others might refer to this as "being in the zone". Regardless, I am certain that you have found it. More importantly, once you do find it, you will unquestionably want to keep it. One thing I have noticed in my years of practicing weight loss management; when finally grasping that success experience, we, as humans, tend to begin a process of fear that it will somehow dissipate, as if it was something rented rather than owned. Not to worry, this feeling is normal. If this is your first time reading this book, you have just begun to scratch the surface of your true potential. Your self-image has unlimited room to grow, but at times, may feel slightly less than stable. You can feel confident that while every single lesson in this book is designed to strengthen your self-image, they are also designed to reinforce and stabilize its growth. Unfortunately, it may be unreasonable to expect you to put every single aspect of this book into practice immediately, and consistently. Luckily, there is one strategy that we have discussed that appears to have stand-alone strength in setting your automatic success mechanism into overdrive.

Just Imagine If...

This one simple recipe, illustrated in Figure 18. A Recipe for Weight Loss Success, for success can have you experiencing success at every turn...just imagine it. Let's take a mixing bowl and blend together a few core ingredients of this book.

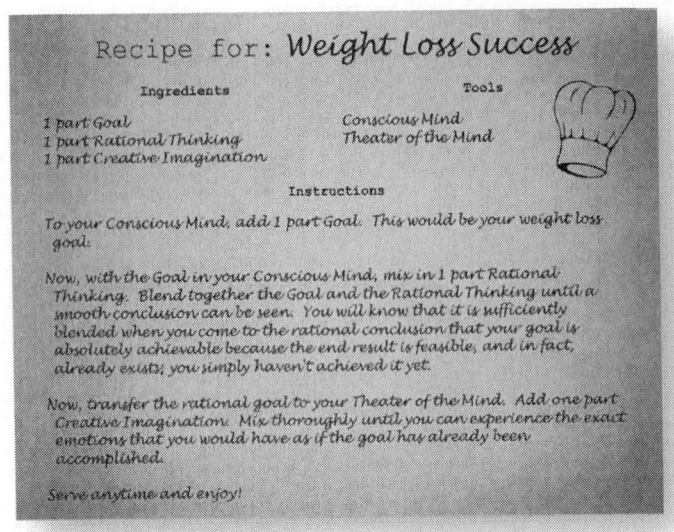

Figure 18. A Recipe for Weight Loss Success

This might seem silly, but there truly is no easier way to generate successful behaviors than by being able to experience the emotions of success on demand. You can access this recipe at any time. Feel free to make this recipe as elaborate and intricate as possible. Add depth and detail to the movie playing out in your mind; the more vivid the details, the greater the emotion that can be evoked from it. Remember, your physical body cannot distinguish between reality and vivid imagination. The emotions will be the same, and "nothing succeeds like success".

It is important to emphasize the reality of this process. Yes, you are "in the zone"; but the zone is not a tangible place. Being in this zone does not warrant you any super powers or magic to yield automatic successful completion of your goal. What it does provide is a sense of drive, desire, and determination to propel you towards your goal. Can you remember that feeling of desire and determination that first day that you started your last diet? Do you remember that feeling of "this time I will succeed", and "I know I can do it"? Of course you do, and like every other attempt that came before it, that feeling dissipated and withered, until you were left with nothing but another failed diet. This recipe can give you that same feeling, every moment of every day, on demand at your beck and call. Now be honest, don't you think this whole process of losing weight can be much, much easier if you had the same drive, desire, and determination everyday as you did on the first day? Maybe even so easy that you could say your weight loss goal is absolutely achievable, with...*Zero Resistance.*

About the Author

Matthew is a Registered Dietitian, practicing with a license in the State of Ohio. Following completion of his undergraduate studies in nutrition and dietetics at Youngstown State University, he went on to receive a Master's of Science of the same concentration at the University of Akron. From there, Matthew completed the esteemed internship at the former Family Health Council of Pittsburgh, now known as Adagio Health. He has been practicing dietetics in the Northeast Ohio area since 2004.

Now residing in his hometown of Youngstown, Ohio, Matthew founded Good Health Industries LLC, an exclusive weight management and obesity reversal professional service, offering unique programs and memberships for clients who have reached the coveted "crisis point" in their lives. Having logged a lifetime of unsuccessful attempts to lose weight, his clients find refuge in his professional knowledge, personal experience, and unbridled compassion for those with the desire of living a healthy life in a body that is comfortable to live it in.

While paying his dues regarding education and professional experience, Matthew attributes the unrivaled success of his clients with his personal familiarity with obesity. From the ages of 18 to 22, Matthew found his weight spiraling out of control, reaching heights of over 330 pounds. Armed with his education, paired with the mindset achieved through the practice of the theses of this book, he was able to regain his self-confidence and achieve a conviction that allowed him to believe in his ability to take charge of his life, losing well over 100 lbs. He has been able to maintain that weight loss for the past decade. Coupling his education, professional experience, and personal history of weight loss success allows Matthew to delve deeper into the unique roots of each of his clients' weight struggles, providing guidance far outreaching that of "calories in versus calories out".

Would you like to learn more about Matthew, Good Health Industries, and the services he provides? Go to ElementsOfGoodHealth.com. Matthew welcomes any and all comments regarding the contents of this book. Comments concerning this book and requests for more information may be directed to info@ElementsOfGoodHealth.com.

Are you ready to send your weight loss journey into overdrive? Just visit members.ElementsOfGoodHealth.com today.

Made in the USA
Lexington, KY
05 December 2013